T0329859

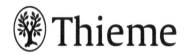

Abbreviated MRI of the Breast

The Practical Guide

Christopher E. Comstock, MD, FACR
Director, Evelyn Lauder Breast Center
Attending Radiologist
Memorial Sloan Kettering Cancer Center
New York, New York

Christiane Kuhl, MD
Professor and Director
Department of Diagnostic and Interventional Radiology
University of Aachen
Aachen, Germany

Thieme
New York • Stuttgart • Delhi • Rio de Janeiro

Thieme Medical Publishers, Inc.
333 Seventh Avenue
New York, New York 10001

Executive Editor: William Lamsback
Managing Editor: J. Owen Zurhellen IV
Editorial Assistant: Mary B. Wilson
Director, Editorial Services: Mary Jo Casey
Production Editor: Sean Woznicki
International Production Director: Andreas Schabert
International Marketing Director: Fiona Henderson
International Sales Director: Louisa Turrell
Director of Sales, North America: Mike Roseman
Senior Vice President and Chief Operating Officer: Sarah Vanderbilt
President: Brian D. Scanlan

Library of Congress Cataloging-in-Publication Data

Names: Comstock, Christopher E., editor. | Kuhl, Christiane, editor.
Title: Abbreviated MRI of the breast : a practical guide / [edited by] Christopher E. Comstock, Christiane Kuhl.
Description: First edition. | New York : Thieme, [2018] | Includes bibliographical references and index.
Identifiers: LCCN 2016049769 (print) | LCCN 2016050230 (ebook)|ISBN 9781626231931 (hardcover : alk. paper)|ISBN 9781626231948 (eBook) | ISBN 9781626231948
Subjects: | MESH: Breast Neoplasms–diagnosis | Magnetic Resonance Imaging–methods
Classification: LCC RC280.B8 (print) | LCC RC280.B8 (ebook) | NLM WP 870 | DDC 616.99/4490754–dc23
LC record available at https://lccn.loc.gov/2016049769

Important note: Medicine is an ever-changing science undergoing continual development. Research and clinical experience are continually expanding our knowledge, in particular our knowledge of proper treatment and drug therapy. Insofar as this book mentions any dosage or application, readers may rest assured that the authors, editors, and publishers have made every effort to ensure that such references are in accordance with **the state of knowledge at the time of production of the book.**

Nevertheless, this does not involve, imply, or express any guarantee or responsibility on the part of the publishers in respect to any dosage instructions and forms of applications stated in the book. **Every user is requested to examine carefully** the manufacturers' leaflets accompanying each drug and to check, if necessary in consultation with a physician or specialist, whether the dosage schedules mentioned therein or the contraindications stated by the manufacturers differ from the statements made in the present book. Such examination is particularly important with drugs that are either rarely used or have been newly released on the market. Every dosage schedule or every form of application used is entirely at the user's own risk and responsibility. The authors and publishers request every user to report to the publishers any discrepancies or inaccuracies noticed. If errors in this work are found after publication, errata will be posted at www.thieme.com on the product description page.

Some of the product names, patents, and registered designs referred to in this book are in fact registered trademarks or proprietary names even though specific reference to this fact is not always made in the text. Therefore, the appearance of a name without designation as proprietary is not to be construed as a representation by the publisher that it is in the public domain.

Thieme Publishers New York
333 Seventh Avenue, New York, NY 10001 USA
+1 800 782 3488, customerservice@thieme.com

Thieme Publishers Stuttgart
Rüdigerstrasse 14, 70469 Stuttgart, Germany
+49 [0]711 8931 421, customerservice@thieme.de

Thieme Publishers Delhi
A-12, Second Floor, Sector-2, Noida-201301
Uttar Pradesh, India
+91 120 45 566 00, customerservice@thieme.in

Thieme Publishers Rio, Thieme Publicações Ltda.
Rua do Matoso 170,
Tijuca, RJ CEP 20270-135
Rio de Janeiro, Brazil
+55 21 2563- 9700

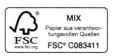

Printed in Germany by CPI books, Leck   5 4 3 2

ISBN 978-1-62623-193-1

Also available as an e-book:
eISBN 978-1-62623-194-8

For Rebecca.

– CEC

For my entire two- and four-legged family.

– CK

Contents

Foreword

When I, accidentally, became involved in breast cancer detection and diagnosis in 1978 (everyone else in the Department of Radiology at the Massachusetts General Hospital refused to read the 8 mammograms that were being performed each day) I firmly believed that someone would discover a cure for breast cancer in the next few years and I would move into a general radiology practice. Now almost 40 years later, there is still no cure for breast cancer. Therapy has improved, but therapy only saves lives when breast cancers are treated before they have become successfully metastatic.

The death rate from breast cancer in the U.S. had been unchanged for at least 50 years (dating back to 1940) until mammography screening was introduced in the mid-1980's. Soon after, in 1990, the death rate began to fall, and as we have continued to improve our ability to detect breast cancers earlier, annual breast cancer deaths have declined by 38% in the U.S. This is a major achievement, but far from victory over the leading cause of non-preventable cancer death (most lung cancers can be prevented) among women. Mammography screening has been a major advance, but 40,000 women still die each year from breast cancer. Many of these deaths are likely due to women not participating in screening, but others are among women for whom mammography screening did not detect their cancers soon enough.

The first randomized, controlled trial of screening asymptomatic women was performed within the Health Insurance Plan of New York (HIP) in the 1960's and showed, for the first time, that earlier detection could not just delay deaths, but could result in cures and eliminate deaths from breast cancer. Tabar's landmark "Swedish Two County" trial showed that major reductions in breast cancer deaths could be accomplished through the use of high-quality mammography screening alone that was able to detect cancers before they were large enough to feel. This led to the start of nationwide screening in the U.S. in the mid-1980's, and in 1990, for the first time in decades, the death rate from breast cancer began to fall and this has continued as more and more women have participated in screening.

The plain industrial film mammograms used in the HIP trial required high doses of x-rays and the quality of the images was poor. Xeroradiography (the fundamental semiconductor technology of today's digital mammograms) resulted in major improvements in detecting breast cancer, and the Breast Cancer Detection Demonstration Project (BCDDP) in the 1970's showed that screening could be efficient and effective in a study that recruited more than 250,000 women across the U.S.

Fluorescent screens were developed for mammography that converted x-rays to light and more efficiently exposed newer film that allowed for still lower dose and improved cancer detection. At around the same time Magnetic Resonance Imaging was being developed for imaging the human body. Initial efforts to apply MRI to the breast were overly optimistic. In the early years intravenous contrast was not available and, although cancers were visible on MRI if they were surrounded by fat, many were hidden by normal fibroglandular tissue, and, in the U.S., interest shifted away from Breast MRI.

The battles to preserve access to breast cancer screening for women ages 40 and over began in the 1970's when screening in the BCDDP was limited by what proved to be false concerns about radiation risk. Even though the scientific evidence showed that lives were saved by screening starting at the age of 40, efforts were increased to try to confine screening to women ages 50 and over. We have thus far been successful in preserving access for women starting at the age of 40 in the U.S., but in Europe, women were, falsely, told that mammography did not save lives until age 50 so that most countries still only encourage screening starting at the age of 50.

While the battle for access to screening has continued, efforts to improve our ability to detect breast cancer before it becomes clinically evident have continued. With the introduction of gadolinium as an intravenous contrast agent the importance of MRI for breast evaluation began to be realized. In my own group at the Massachusetts General Hospital, Priscilla Slanetz studied women with recently discovered breast cancer who volunteered to have a research MRI with gadolinium and, in 1997, she began to find unexpected cancers in the opposite breast that were not visible by mammography. Although the publication of her work was held up for two years, she was among the first (if not the first) to show that MRI could detect breast cancers in "normal breasts" that were not evident on film/screen mammograms. For the first time, it became clear to us that MRI could represent a valuable "second level" screening test to find cancers that were not evident by mammography.

Over the same period digital detectors were finally developed for mammography, delayed by the unique FDA requirement that they undergo an expensive premarket approval process (PMA) unlike the adoption of digital for bone, abdomen, chest, etc. which only had to pass the simpler and much less expensive 510K requirements. Despite some convoluted analyses, Full Field Digital Mammography (FFDM) did not really increase our ability to detect breast cancers, but digital provided improvements in the logistics of mammography, and, more importantly, opened new opportunities for the use of x-rays. Having access to an early digital detector, I invented, and my group at the MGH developed Digital Breast Tomosynthesis (DBT) which has become a major advance in breast cancer screening by detecting more breast cancers at a small and curable size while reducing the recall rate (pejoratively called "false positives").

At the same time more and more effort was going into improving MRI for breast evaluation. Even as we were developing DBT, it became clear that the absolutely single best way to find the most breast cancers earlier was by using MRI with gadolinium contrast enhancement to take advantage of the neovascularity that all breast cancers require to grow larger than a few millimeters. MRI has become, far and away, the single best way to find small invasive breast cancers. However, in addition to the high cost of MRI, it has been, falsely argued, that the cancers it was finding are likely not "real" breast cancers because they are found at a rate that is much higher than the rate that clinically evident masses ("real cancers") are found each year. In his introductory chapter Dr. Comstock has provided the explanation. What most do not realize is that breast cancers do not grow from a single cell to a 2 cm. mass in one year. In fact, if the average doubling time for a breast cancer is 120 days, it may take 20 years for the first cancer cell to multiply to a 2 cm. mass. This means that, in order to have 1-5 breast cancers become clinically evident each year among women ages 40 and over, there has to be a huge reservoir (many times this number) of smaller cancers growing in the population "beneath the surface". This fact was reinforced in what was, essentially, a random sample of the number of breast cancers in a population of women, with a study from the four corners region of the U.S. in which the breasts of women who died accidentally were autopsied. The investigators discovered 11 cancers among 500 wom-

en. This rate of 22 cancers per 1000 women supports the fact that there are many more cancers growing in the population to sustain the 1-5 each year that become clinically evident. These are "real" cancers that are growing and will develop metastatic potential as they increase in size.

It is clear that MRI is the best way to find many if not most of these cancers. There are certainly some extremely small breast cancers that are metastatic (and incurable) before they can be detected, and some very large cancers that are indolent, but the smaller the cancer the less likely it has become successfully metastatic and the more likely it can be cured. Given the fact that death from breast cancer still correlates in large part with the size of the cancer when it is removed, it is likely that detecting these, almost universally small, breast cancers using MRI, will further reduce deaths.

One other fact that is critical is that, although research has uncovered the genetic mutations that are associated with women who are at very high risk of developing breast cancer, these only account for, at most, 10% of the women who are diagnosed each year. The vast majority of women (75%) who are diagnosed with breast cancer each year are among women who have none of the known elevators of risk. For many years, screening using MRI, despite its major advantages over everything else, has been too expensive to be used in the general population and has been confined to screening only high risk women. It is women who are at average risk for developing breast cancer who account for most of the cases each year and who need to participate in screening.

I remember over the years looking at the Maximum Intensity Projection (MIP) of the pre and post contrast MR images and seeing how clearly the cancer was seen, but then dutifully looking at all the other pulse sequences that we had collected (accounting for most of the scan time) never thinking that they were fairly superfluous for the vast majority of scans. It was not until Dr. Kuhl realized that if MRI was to be used for screening, to efficiently evaluate a huge number of women to find the few that needed additional evaluation and harbored the cancers, all that was needed was this MIP!! As with so many important discoveries it took someone to realize its value. By reducing the scan time to only a few minutes it becomes economically feasible to apply MRI as a screening test for "average risk" women.

Therapy for breast cancer has improved. Therapy can delay many deaths, but if breast cancer is successfully metastatic it cannot be cured. Although mammography screening has reduced the death rate by 38%, Drs. Comstock, Kuhl and the other Breast MRI experts who have authored this timely text now offer the opportunity to dramatically drive down deaths. By using this greatly shortened protocol it becomes possible to screen the general population with MRI. This may actually head us toward curing many if not most breast cancers. I congratulate Drs. Comstock and Kuhl for their excellent textbook that may well mark the beginning of the end of breast cancer as a major killer, and I will finally be able to pursue a career in general radiology!

Daniel B. Kopans, MD, FACR
Founder – Breast Imaging Division
Massachusetts General Hospital
Professor of Radiology
Harvard Medical School
Boston, Massachusetts

Preface

Breast cancer continues to represent the most frequent type of cancer diagnosed in the female population. In spite of several decades of publicly organized mammographic screening programs, breast cancer continues to represent the first (several European countries) or second (United States) most important cause of cancer death in the female population. It is time to search for other improved breast cancer screening methods.

Over the last decades, it has become increasingly evident that breast MRI offers a substantially higher sensitivity and thus improves early diagnosis of breast cancer compared to screening mammography – irrespective of the type of breast cancer, irrespective of its local stage, irrespective of whether it is invasive or intraductal, irrespective whether it is primary or recurrent, and irrespective of a woman's breast density, her family history or overall breast cancer risk. Accordingly, MRI is the imaging method of choice when it comes to breast cancer screening – if there weren't the cost and greatly limited availability of this method in contemporary clinical medicine. The concept of abbreviated breast MRI may be the missing link to help us overcome these limitations and potentially change the current standards of practice.

This is the first textbook dedicated on the subject of AB-MR. In this book, we provide fundamental guidelines for radiologists for implementing, performing and interpreting AB-MR. We provide a background of AB-MR, including a review of current research data as well as technical approaches that have been successfully pursued, provide information on accurate interpretation in a flow chart format, and techniques for biopsy, all of which may be used by both American and international radiologists specializing in breast imaging. The editors of this book are the principle investigators in the first multicenter trial evaluating AB-MR and the authors of each chapter are leaders in the field of breast MRI, and are therefore able to offer a unique and practical approach to AB-MR.

We hope that this book will foster the rapid dissemination of abbreviated breast MRI, and, increase access to the most powerful tool for early diagnosis of breast cancer that we currently have. With AB-MR, we have the opportunity to fundamentally change how women are screened for breast cancer. The information in this book will allow radiologists throughout the world to be better prepared as we enter this new era in breast cancer screening.

Acknowledgments

We thank Dr. Janice Sung not only for her co-authored chapters but also for her editing and significant contribution to several other chapters. In addition she has been a vital behind-the-scenes contributor to the development and approval process of the EA1141 AB-MR multicenter trial that is now open and accruing.

Contributors

Christopher E. Comstock, MD
Director, Evelyn Lauder Breast Center
Attending Radiologist
Memorial Sloan Kettering Cancer Center
New York, New York

R. Edward Hendrick, PhD, FACR
Clinical Professor
Department of Radiology
University of Colorado–Denver
Aurora, Colorado

Christiane Kuhl, MD
Professor and Director
Department of Diagnostic and Interventional
   Radiology
University of Aachen
Aachen, Germany

Carol H. Lee, MD
Diagnostic Radiologist
Memorial Sloan Kettering Cancer Center
New York, New York

Constance D. Lehman, MD, PhD, FACR
Director of Cancer Imaging
Department of Radiology
University of Washington
Seattle, Washington

Elizabeth A. Morris, MD
Chief, Breast Imaging Service
Larry Norton Chair
Memorial Sloan Kettering Cancer Center
New York, New York

Gillian M. Newstead, MD, FACR
Department of Radiology
University of Chicago
Chicago, Illinois

Janice S. Sung, MD
Radiologist
Memorial Sloan Kettering Cancer Center
New York, New York

1 Introduction to Abbreviated Breast Magnetic Imaging

Christopher E. Comstock

1.1 Introduction

It is time for a fundamental change in how we screen women for breast cancer. For the past 40 years, mammography has been the primary test used to screen for breast cancer. To date, mammography is the only imaging modality that has been shown in multiple randomized controlled clinical trials and observational studies to reduce the number of deaths from breast cancer.[1,2,3] Breast cancer mortality is decreased by approximately 30% when women are screened with mammography. With the widespread adoption of screening mammography in the United States in the mid-1980s, a subsequent decrease in mortality became apparent beginning in the 1990s.[4] However, despite mammographic screening, approximately 40,000 women continue to die from breast cancer each year. During the entire 10 years of the Vietnam War, a total of 47,424 U.S. combat soldiers died, resulting in massive antiwar demonstrations and the eventual withdrawal of U.S. troops. A similar number of women die each year from breast cancer; where is the national outrage?

Approximately 30,000 people die in motor vehicle accidents each year in the United States. In an effort to reduce fatalities, we have seen dramatic advancements in auto safety technology such as the development of air bags as well as collision avoidance, lane assist, drowsy driver detection, and auto piloting systems. More women die each year from breast cancer than from car accidents. Major technological advances have been seen throughout all sectors of society in the past half-century including military, aeronautic, satellite, and computer technologies. However, mammography as well as our approach to breast cancer screening has remained relatively unchanged for the past 50 years (▶ Fig. 1.1).

Although mammography is an effective screening test, it is a suboptimal test. A mammogram is a two-dimensional (2D) image (or shadow) of the breast and its sensitivity is limited by breast density. This is a major limitation of screening mammography given that approximately 50% of women in the United States have heterogeneously or extremely dense breasts. In addition, the average tumor size of a cancer detected on a screening mammogram is 1.4 cm and approximately 20% of screen-detected cancers have axillary nodal metastases. Another limitation of mammography is the interval cancer rate; 20% of all breast cancers are interval cancers, meaning that these cancers are diagnosed within 365 days of having a negative mammogram. Interval cancers also tend to be more aggressive and are associated with a worse prognosis. Additional limitations of mammography include the recall rate and false-positive biopsy rate. Approximately 10% of women are recalled after a screening mammogram for further evaluation of a questionable finding; in the majority of cases, no suspicious abnormality is seen when additional mammographic views and/or ultrasound are performed. Finally, when a biopsy is recommended for a mammographic lesion, approximately 70% of those are found to be benign.

Attempts have been made to improve mammographic technology in order to address some of these limitations. These include the conversion from industrial to high-speed screen film, computer-aided detection (CAD) programs, digital mammography, and now digital breast tomosynthesis (DBT). Industrial film was initially used in screening mammography. With time, analog films evolved first to the use of film with grids, then to the use of screen film combinations, and then to high-speed film. The development of high-speed, high-contrast film improved image quality and image consistency. CAD programs were developed in the 1990s in order to highlight areas on the mammogram that may be abnormal. The primary goal of CAD programs is to increase cancer detection, reducing the number of false negatives. Digital mammography was another advancement that was developed in early 2000s. With digital technique, the degree of image contrast can be adjusted to optimize visualization even in areas of dense breast tissue. The Digital Mammographic Imaging Screening Trial (DMIST) was a prospective multicenter trial that included 49,528 women. The trial was designed as a comparative study, with all women undergoing both digital and film mammography in random order. In DMIST, the accuracy of digital mammography was significantly higher than film mammography in women under the age of 50, women with heterogeneously or extremely dense breasts, and in premenopausal or perimenopausal women.

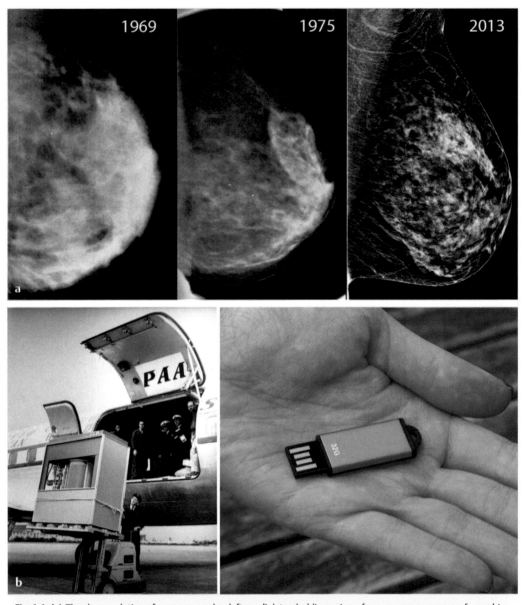

Fig. 1.1 (a) The slow evolution of mammography: left mediolateral oblique views from mammograms performed in 1969, 1975, and 2013. **(b)** Yet computer memory, for example, has progressed from a 1.5-ton hard drive of 5 megabytes in 1956 (left) to today's inexpensive USB flash drives with thousands of times the capacity and weighing just a few grams (right).

DBT was Food and Drug Administration (FDA) approved in 2011 and is the latest attempt to improve the sensitivity and specificity of mammography. DBT obtains a series of low-dose mammograms at varies angles in order to reconstruct 3D images of the breast. DBT is slowly replacing conventional 2D full-field digital mammogram (FFDM) at many centers throughout the United States. Multiple large studies have demonstrated that when DBT is used in addition to a standard 2D FFDM, the cancer detection rate is increased by 0.7 to 2.7 cancers per 1,000 women.[5,6,7,8,9] Another benefit of DBT besides increased sensitivity is that the number of women asked to return for additional imaging is reduced by approximately 15% as the tomosynthesis images help decrease unnecessary callbacks due to summation of overlapping normal tissue.[5,6,7,8,9]

Despite these advances in mammographic technique, the cancer detection rate is only slightly improved. Screening mammography still relies on trying to distinguish cancers from the surrounding normal fibroglandular tissue based on a 2D morphological signal or shadow.

Magnetic resonance imaging (MRI) is a vascular-based test not limited by breast density. It has long been known to be the most sensitive test for breast cancer detection, but its use has been restricted to women at the highest risk for breast cancer primarily due to its high cost, time to perform, and perceived low positive predictive value (PPV). However, the landscape of breast cancer screening has changed due to the passage of breast density legislation (BDL) in many states. Many women with mammographically dense breasts are now screened with a combination of both mammography and whole breast ultrasound. An abbreviated breast MRI (AB-MR) that is more sensitive and specific than mammography and ultrasound with a comparable cost may be a more effective way to screen women with dense breasts for breast cancer. However, in order to understand the potential of AB-MR in this new role, it is important to understand the principles of breast cancer screening, what we have learned from BDL, and factors to consider in successfully implementing an AB-MR screening program.

1.2 Principles of Breast Cancer Screening

Outside of minor fluctuations in breast cancer rates over time due to dietary and environmental factors as well as aging of the population, women develop breast cancer at a relatively constant rate. In the absence of screening tests, these cancers will present as palpable masses once they reach a certain size. The use of a screening test allows some cancers to be detected earlier, at a smaller size before they are palpable. Although the total number of cancers detected remains the same, with screening, the combination of the screen-detected cancers and fewer palpable cancers results in a smaller average tumor size and stage at detection. This translates into a reduction in mortality and the use of less aggressive therapies. The average size of cancers detected and the ratio of screen detected to palpable (interval) cancers is directly related to the performance of the screening technology (▶ Fig. 1.2).

Reported sensitivities of a screening test can be very misleading and are dependent on what is being used as the reference standard for the test. For example, although the sensitivity of mammography has been reported as 60 to 80% based on a reference standard of 1 year of follow-up, the true sensitivity based on the number of cancers

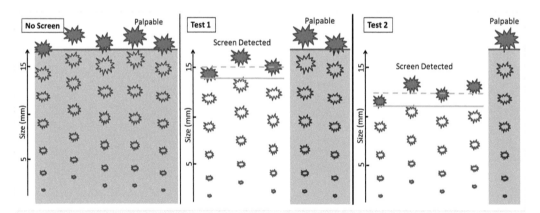

Fig. 1.2 Comparing the performance of two screening tests. In this example, without screening, a total of five cancers develop and are detected only as palpable masses. With screening, some of these same five cancers will be detected by the screening test at a smaller size before they are palpable. With Test 1, three cancers are detected with a mean size of 1.5 cm. However, two cancers are missed on this screening test and will present as palpable interval cancers, resulting in a sensitivity of 60%. Test 2 is a more sensitive test, and detected four of five cancers (sensitivity of 80%). Test 2 also detects cancers at a smaller size than Test 1 with a mean size of 1.2 cm. Only one cancer will present as a palpable interval cancer. Although there are a total of five cancers in both groups, Test 2 detects the cancers at a smaller size with fewer interval (palpable) cancers than test 1. By detecting cancers at a smaller size and earlier stage, Test 2 results in a greater reduction in breast cancer mortality and morbidity.

mammography detects out of the total number of cancers present in the women at the time of the test (reservoir of cancers) is significantly less. A single round of MRI in 1,000 women with a negative mammogram has been shown to find 15 or more additional cancers. Mammography detects approximately 5 to 6 cancers per 1,000 women out of the 20 or so cancers that could be detected with combined screening with mammography and MRI. Therefore, the sensitivity of mammography based on this reference standard is only 30% or less. The reservoir of breast cancers present in women is undoubtedly higher than 20 cancers per 1,000 women. A test that could find cancers at its earliest stage at a size of 1 mm or even less could theoretically reveal a reservoir of cancers on the order of 50 to 100 cancers per 1,000 women (▶ Fig. 1.3). This would show the sensitivities of current breast cancer screening tests to be significantly lower than reported.

The first round of screening is referred to as the prevalence screen. On the prevalence screen, more cancers will be found because the screening test will detect cancers in the reservoir which have reached the lower threshold set by the screening test that otherwise would have later presented as palpable masses. On subsequent screening rounds (incidence screens), the cancer detection rate will return to the same rate as it was prior to the institution of screening. The only difference is that once breast cancer screening is instituted, the cancer reservoir will be smaller and subsequent cancers will be detected at a smaller average size and stage, with fewer becoming palpable or clinically evident. Debating the precise benefits of breast cancer screening and rehashing the various randomized control screening trials is beyond the scope of this book. Our assumption and belief is that finding breast cancer at a smaller size and earlier stage will reduce morbidity and mortality from breast cancer, just as screening does for colon, skin, cervical, and other cancers (▶ Table 1.1).

Breast cancer screening programs and how they are designed to lower the reservoir of cancers in women are somewhat arbitrary. They depend on the technologies available and what is considered acceptable in terms of cost, time, test frequency, and false positives versus the number and stage of cancers that are detected. In addition, what the scientific community considers appropriate for a breast screening program may not always coincide with what the public wants. This is evident by the proliferation of BDL across many states in which women with dense breasts have demanded the addition of ultrasound to screening mammography in order to detect a few additional cancers despite the relatively poor performance, high cost,

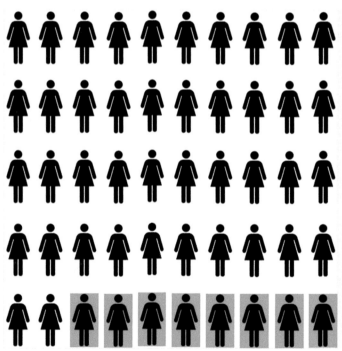

Fig. 1.3 Reservoir of breast cancers. The number of cancers present in 1,000 women being screened at a given time is unknown. Combined screening with mammography and ultrasound will detect approximately 7 to 8 cancers per 1,000 women. An additional 14 cancers will be detected on the first round of screening magnetic resonance imaging.

Table 1.1 Impact of tumor size on breast cancer mortality

Tumor size	Relative risk
Carcinoma in situ	0.41
1–9 mm	1.0
10–14 mm	1.58
15–19 mm	2.71
20–29 mm	4.88
30–49 mm	8.92
≥ 50 mm	19.00

Adapted from László Tabár, Bedrich Vitak, Hsiu-Hsi Chen, Stephen W. Duffy, Ming-Fang Yen, Ching-Feng Chiang, Ulla Brith Krusemo, Tibor Tot, Robert A. Smith. The Swedish Two-Country Trial Twenty Years Later: Updated Mortality Results and New Insights from Long-Term Follow-up. Radiologic Clinics of North America, Volume 38, Issue 4, 2000, 625–651

and increased false positives of screening ultrasound. Our current approach to reducing the reservoir of breast cancers in women is to combine annual mammography with annual whole breast screening ultrasound (WBUS) which results in an approximate detection rate of 8 cancers per 1,000 average risk women screened. Is there a more efficient way to detect more breast cancers at a smaller size, lower cost, and with fewer false positives? In addition, are there screening technologies that can find cancers that are more biologically significant or harmful?

1.3 The Current Landscape of Breast Cancer Screening

For over 40 years, mammography has been the primary modality used for breast cancer screening. Screening mammography is the only imaging test shown to decrease mortality from breast cancer. A randomized control trial (RCT) is the most rigorous type of study to determine whether a screening test is effective. In terms of screening mammography, there have been eight major RCTs. In these RCTs, an approximate 30% decrease in breast cancer mortality was seen following the institution of screening mammography. The RCTs have also demonstrated that a mortality reduction is likely to be seen approximately 5 to 7 years after the onset of screening mammography.

The performance and limitations of a screening test are directly related to the physical properties used by the test to detect cancer. One limitation of mammography, since it is based on the penetration and resolution of X-rays to discern structures in the breast based on morphology, is that its sensitivity is affected by breast density. The fifth edition of the Breast Imaging Reporting and Data System (BIRADS) categorizes breast density as almost entirely fatty, scattered areas of fibroglandular density, heterogeneously dense and extremely dense.[10] A woman is considered to have dense breasts if mammographically her density is categorized as either heterogeneously dense or extremely dense. Data from the Breast Cancer Surveillance Consortium (BCSC), which reviewed over 900,000 mammograms, revealed that 46.9% of women have mammographically dense breasts.[11]

Breast density is important because of its effect on both the accuracy of screening mammography and its association with increased breast cancer risk. Normal fibroglandular tissue appears dense mammographically, and obscures visualization of cancers, which also are radiodense. The sensitivity of film screen mammography decreased from 85.7% to 88.8% in women with almost entirely fatty breasts to 62.2% to 68.1% in women with extremely dense breasts.[12,13] Sensitivity of mammography in women with dense breasts has improved with the development of digital mammography. In the DMIST trial, the sensitivity of digital mammography in women with dense breasts was 70%, compared to 55% in film screen mammography.[14]

There is also an association between having mammographically dense breasts and increased breast cancer risk. Boyd et al reported that in 1,112 matched case–control pairs, women with extremely dense breasts were 4.7 times more likely to develop breast cancer than patients with < 10% fibroglandular density.[15] Another meta-analysis, which included data from over 240,000 mammograms from 42 studies, reported a relative risk of 2.92 for breasts that are 50 to 75% dense and a relative risk of 4.64 for breasts that are at least 75% dense.[16] In many studies, the relative risk of women with extremely dense breasts is compared to women with almost entirely fat density, which are the two extremes of the population. Only approximately 10% of women in the United States have predominantly fatty breasts and another 10% have extremely dense breasts. When compared to women with average breast density, the relative risk is reduced to 1.2 for heterogeneously dense breasts and 2.1 for extremely dense breasts.[17] Finally, several studies have shown that the association of dense breasts and breast cancer is not due to the masking effect alone.[15,18,19]

Due to the increasing public awareness of the shortcomings of mammography, in 2009 Connecticut became the first state to pass BDL. Many states followed and breast density notification laws are now in effect in 27 states. These laws require that women be notified if they are found to have mammographically dense breasts. In some states, the legislation also specifies that women be told some or all of the following: that mammography may be less sensitive for breast cancer detection in women with dense breasts, that dense breast tissue may increase a woman's risk for breast cancer, and that supplemental screening should be considered. However, most states do not mandate insurance coverage of supplemental screening.

These laws impact a very large number of women; more than 50% of women younger than 50 years and at least 33% of women older than 50 have dense breasts.[20] In addition, nearly 65% of women in the United States live in states that have enacted BDL. Although the density legislation does not mandate the specific type of supplemental screening test women should consider, WBUS has become the default supplemental screening test. WBUS is a relatively inexpensive test to perform, widely available, and familiar to patients. This has led to a dramatic increase in the utilization of breast ultrasound. The primary advantage of WBUS is that it detects additional cancers that are mammographically occult in 2 to 4 per 1,000 women. Most cancers detected on WBUS are invasive, node negative cancers that are approximately 1 cm in size. However, significant limitations of WBUS include a recall rate of up to 20% and a PPV of approximately 8%.[21,22,23] Therefore, 12 benign biopsies are performed before 1 cancer is detected on a screening breast ultrasound. WBUS is also time-consuming for technologist and radiologists and leads to a significant number of short-term follow-up recommendations. WBUS in women with dense breasts has also been shown in modeling studies not to be cost-effective, substantially increasing health care costs while providing small benefits.[23]

The landscape of breast cancer screening is no longer based solely on mortality data from RCTs and academic assertion on what is acceptable in terms of time, cost, and possible harms of screening, but also on grassroots movements and public opinion on what efforts should be taken to find a woman's breast cancer at its earliest stages. Because of this, for many women, the current landscape of breast cancer screening has evolved from annual mammography to a program of annual mammography combined with annual WBUS. Now that these new expectations on our screening program have been set forth, our goal is to improve the cancer detection process by reducing the inefficiencies, cost, and false positives while finding biologically significant cancers at a smaller size and stage and reducing interval cancers.

1.4 Concept of Abbreviated Breast Magnetic Resonance Imaging

Breast MRI is currently the most sensitive test for detecting breast cancer. Screening mammography detects approximately 4 to 6 cancers per 1,000 women screened. With WBUS, an additional 2 to 4 mammographically occult cancers per 1,000 women are detected. However, several studies have demonstrated that breast MRI can detect a substantially larger reservoir of breast cancers that are mammographically and sonographically occult. For example, in the ACRIN 6666 trial, a screening breast MRI was performed in women with dense breasts. A single MRI performed in women after three rounds of negative screening mammograms and ultrasound detected an additional 14.7 cancers per 1,000.[24] Importantly, the PPV3 of MRI was 23% compared to 9 to 11.7% for WBUS. Another study included 427 asymptomatic women at mild to moderately increased risk for breast cancer and dense breasts. In these women with a negative FFDM and WBUS, screening MRI resulted in an additional cancer yield of 18.2 per 1,000.[25] There were seven invasive cancers (64%) and four cases (36%) of ductal carcinoma in situ (DCIS). The invasive cancers detected were small T1, node negative cancers, and both the invasive cancers and DCIS were predominantly high-grade tumors. WBUS in the 11 patients diagnosed with breast cancer was negative.

These studies demonstrate that there is a large reservoir of cancers in the breast that are not detected on either screening mammography or ultrasound, and that there is a technology (MRI) available that is able to detect these cancers at a smaller size and stage compared to either mammography or WBUS without sacrificing specificity. However, due to its high cost, time to perform, perceived low PPV3, and limited availability, screening MRI has been restricted to a small select group of extremely high-risk women. How can we expand the use of MRI to benefit more women?

1.5 It Is Time for a Fundamental Change in How We Utilize MRI for Breast Cancer Screening

The performance of breast MRI has not changed significantly in almost 20 years, with standard protocols including a localizer, T2 weighted with or without fat saturation, a T1 precontrast non–fat-saturated, and a precontrast and multiple dynamic postcontrast T1 weighted sequence. In general, the scan time of a typical breast MRI ranges from 20 to 40 minutes, and patients are scheduled in 45- to 60-minute slots. As currently used, it would not be feasible to expand the role of breast MRI to screen a broader population, such as all women with dense breasts.

What would make MRI screening more feasible? MRI would need to be more efficient with a similar cost and time to perform compared to current practice (e.g., mammography and WBUS in women with dense breasts). Given reimbursement rates in general, a breast MRI would need to be performed within approximately 10 minutes to be comparable in cost to a WBUS. The concept of an AB-MR is to reduce the time to perform the study by including only the most essential sequences while maintaining sensitivity and specificity. Most of the sensitivity and diagnostic information is captured in the first postcontrast series, including lesion morphology and rate of early enhancement. Removing the additional postcontrast dynamic series primarily impacts evaluation of lesion kinetics. Kinetic information is utilized relatively infrequently, such as when deciding to recommend biopsy or follow-up of a lesion on a baseline MR. A T2 weighted sequence is more valuable in breast MR interpretation to improve specificity on a baseline MR. On subsequent screening rounds after a baseline study, kinetic and T2 signal provide little additional information given development of a new or enlarging enhancing lesion is most predictive of malignancy, irrespective of its kinetics and T2 signal. Therefore, an AB-MR protocol that includes a localizer, a T2 weighted sequence, and a T1 weighted sequence before and after contrast administration would allow sites to expand the use of screening MRI to more women without

significantly impacting its performance compared to a traditional full MRI.

Given the poor performance of combined mammography and WBUS in terms of false positives and short-term follow-up recommendations, an AB-MR program may be more cost-effective (▶ Table 1.2). The difference in the cost of screening with AB-MR versus WBUS will depend on the local reimbursement rate and the payer mix. With an AB-MR costing in the range of $300 to $400, annual screening with AB-MR would likely cost more than WBUS. This cost may be justified due to the increased cancer detection rate of AB-MR, reduced interval cancer rate, and detection of smaller and earlier stage cancers. As MRI detects more than double the number of cancers found on mammography combined with WBUS, AB-MR may only need to be performed biennially to have similar or better performance to annual screening with combined mammography and WBUS. Biennial screening with AB-MR would cost less than annual screening with WBUS.

MRI also has been shown to preferentially detect intermediate and high-grade cancers, which are more likely to be biologically significant[26] (▶ Fig. 1.4). Since screening trials using mortality as an endpoint are impractical due to the time and costs involved, trials of newer modalities such as digital mammography, tomosynthesis, and WBUS have used the number of breast cancers detected as a surrogate endpoint to mortality. However, the biological detection profile of cancers may be more significant compared to just the number of cancers detected. Detecting more biologically significant cancers may decrease mortality while reducing overdiagnosis and overtreatment.

1.6 Successful Implementation of an AB-MR Program

Much can be learned from the history of mammography and its eventual adoption. Despite the introduction of mammography for breast cancer screening in the 1930s, and further technological improvements by Robert Egan in the 1950s, mammography languished until the 1970s. This shows us that improvements in medical technology and image resolution are not the sole driving forces in acceptance and widespread clinical adoption of a screening test. Mammography only became accepted once various economic, social, political, and scientific barriers were overcome. The adoption of mammography only occurred in

Table 1.2 Cost comparison of WBUS and AB-MR per 1,000 women screened

	Annual WBUS	$300 annual AB-MR	$350 annual AB-MR	$350 biennial AB-MR
Screening exam	182,250	300,000	350,000	175,000
Callback for diagnostic US	9,112.5	N/A	N/A	
Second look US after MR	NA	3,000	3,500	2,625
Six-month follow-up exams	18,225	15,000	17,500	12,250
US biopsy	41,324	8,264.8	8,264.8	5,785.36
MR biopsy	NA	50,786.8	50,786.8	35,298.76
Pathology	13,450	13,450	13,450	6,725
US cyst-guided aspiration	1,565	N/A	N/A	N/A
Total	265,926.5	390,501.6	443,501.60	237,684.12
Total per women screened	265.92	390.50	443.50	237.68

Abbreviations: AB-MR, abbreviated breast magnetic resonance imaging; US, ultrasound; WBUS, whole breast screening ultrasound.
Assumptions: Payer mix of 55% Medicare and 45% private insurance, and a private insurance reimbursement rate of 1.28 × Medicare rate.
Twenty percent of biopsies are performed in a hospital-based setting and 80% in freestanding centers.
Callback rate for diagnostic US from WBUS: 5%.
Ultrasound BI-RADS 3 rate: 10%.
MR BI-RADS 3 rate: 5%.
Ultrasound cyst aspirate rate: 1%.
Ultrasound biopsy rate: 5%.
MR targeted ultrasound rate: 1%.
MR biopsy rate: 5%.
For biennial AB-MR, MR targeted US rate, MR BI-RADS 3, and MR biopsy rates increase to 1.5, 7, and 7%, respectively.

the context of the 1971 Health Insurance Plan (HIP) randomized controlled trial demonstrating that screening mammography decreased breast cancer mortality, the American Cancer Society's public war on cancer emphasizing the role of mammography as a weapon against breast cancer, and the emergence of breast imaging as a subspecialty of radiology in the late 1960s.[27]

The widespread adoption of AB-MR for breast cancer screening in women with dense breasts will require similar acceptance on multiple fronts. MRI has already been established as a technological advancement over mammography and ultrasound. The passage of BDL in numerous states demonstrates that the socioeconomic climate is open to AB-MR. The results of the multicenter Eastern Cooperative Oncology Group (ECOG)—American College of Radiology Imaging Network (ACRIN) study comparing AB-MR to DBT (EA1141) may provide further scientific data to promote widespread acceptance of AB-MR. The trial will not only compare the cancer detection rates between the two modalities on the incidence screen (baseline), but also evaluate the interval cancer rate, differences in tumor biologies, and their performance on the subsequent prevalence screen.

Successful implementation will require increased access to MRI across the country, including rural centers. Companies are currently developing dedicated, less expensive breast magnets in the range of $500,000. This would allow breast centers to operate their own MRI rather than having to share time on general-purpose magnets. In addition, the number of trained MR technologists will need to increase in order to fulfill the growing demand. To simplify the process, companies are exploring "one

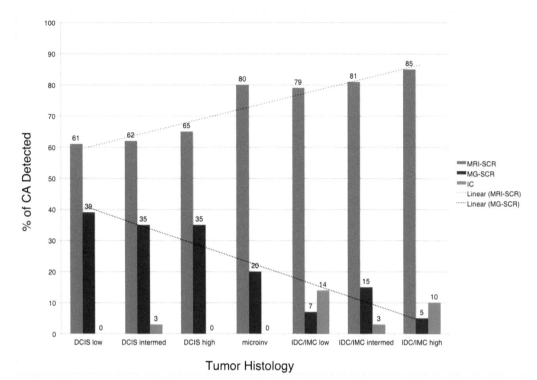

Fig. 1.4 Comparison of tumor histologies by method of detection. Magnetic resonance imaging (MRI) is more sensitive than mammography for all tumor histologies, but especially invasive cancers. More than 80% of intermediate- and high-grade invasive cancers are detected on screening MRI and not mammography in women undergoing combined screening. CA, cancer; DCIS, ductal carcinoma in situ; microinv, microinvasive cancer; IDC, invasive ductal carcinoma; IMC, invasive mammary carcinoma.[26]

touch" scanning where all parameters are automated and detachable ergonomic tables to allow faster positioning and patient throughput. Although AB-MR requires intravenous access for contrast administration, this should not deter women given that many blood tests have become a routine part of yearly medical exams, such as screening for cholesterol or diabetes and other screening tests. There has been concern recently regarding possible effects of repeated gadolinium exposure and deposition in the brain. At this point, this has only been an observation and no cellular pathology or clinical symptoms have been attributed to the gadolinium deposition. Companies are performing considerable research to understand the agents prone to cause this, how gadolinium disassociates from its chelate, and to explore new potential contrast agents.

An important component to maintaining high quality and patient satisfaction is the concept of socially responsible imaging. This would include a high level of quality assurance, standardized interpretation, and reader training and certification.

The Society of Breast MRI has established interpretation guidelines, reader training, and an interpretation test specifically for AB-MR. In addition, sites should also participate in tumor registries to monitor the performance of AB-MR nationally. Finally, because comparison to prior MRIs is critical in reducing false positives, file transfer or cloud services should be provided to connect sites to ensure that a patient's prior studies are easily accessible regardless of the location they were performed.

1.7 Future Directions

Annual mammographic screening supplemented by AB-MR every 1 to 3 years, depending on a patient's risk, may be more efficient and effective than mammography supplemented by WBUS in women with dense breasts. The definition of AB-MR is somewhat arbitrary. Local reimbursement rates will likely determine the number and types of sequences that can be performed for AB-MR to yield a similar hourly reimbursement rate that is comparable to full breast MRI. At many centers, a standard full breast MRI protocol can already be completed in 15 to 20 minutes or less. However, without a specific billing code for AB-MR, sites are reluctant to offer AB-MR for fear of having their reimbursement for full breast MRI cut. Widespread adoption of AB-MR will only occur when it has been firmly established as superior to WBUS and public demand forces administrators to change how we utilize MRI for patient care. In the end, establishment of AB-MR will change the current mindset that MRI should be restricted to only a small select group of high-risk women. Widespread utilization of breast MRI will eventually lead to competition in the marketplace. In order to compete, centers will begin to include additional sequences in their AB-MR protocol in order to maximize sensitivity and specificity. In addition, with increasing revenues from breast MRI and competition for market share, companies will strive to improve diffusion weighted imaging, spectroscopy, and noncontrast imaging techniques. Much needed improvements in breast MRI workstation readout through computer-assisted detection and diagnosis and standardized interpretation will also occur. Finally, vascular-based imaging such as MRI may prove to be not only more efficient in detecting breast cancers than mammography plus WBUS but also more selective in detecting the biologically significant tumors. It is surprising how long we have underutilized a test that detects three times as many cancers as mammography. We are on the verge of a fundamental change in how we screen women for breast cancer. Eventually AB-MR may be used as a stand-alone breast cancer screening test performed every few years, replacing annual mammography and WBUS altogether.

References

[1] Tabár L, Vitak B, Chen TH, et al. Swedish two-county trial: impact of mammographic screening on breast cancer mortality during 3 decades. Radiology. 2011; 260(3):658–663

[2] Alexander FE, Anderson TJ, Brown HK, et al. 14 years of follow-up from the Edinburgh randomised trial of breast-cancer screening. Lancet. 1999; 353(9168):1903–1908

[3] Bjurstam N, Björneld L, Warwick J, et al. The Gothenburg Breast Screening Trial. Cancer. 2003; 97(10):2387–2396

[4] Surveillance Epidemiology and End Results (SEER) Program. SEER*Stat Database: Mortality—All COD, Aggregated with County, Total U.S. (1969–2010)<Katrina/Rita population adjustment>—Linked to County Attributes—Total U.S. Available at: http://www.seer.cancer.gov

[5] Ciatto S, Houssami N, Bernardi D, et al. Integration of 3D digital mammography with tomosynthesis for population breast-cancer screening (STORM): a prospective comparison study. Lancet Oncol. 2013; 14(7):583–589

[6] Skaane P, Bandos AI, Gullien R, et al. Prospective trial comparing full-field digital mammography (FFDM) versus combined FFDM and tomosynthesis in a population-based screening programme using independent double reading with arbitration. Eur Radiol. 2013; 23(8):2061–2071

[7] Rose SL, Tidwell AL, Bujnoch LJ, Kushwaha AC, Nordmann AS, Sexton R, Jr. Implementation of breast tomosynthesis in a routine screening practice: an observational study. AJR Am J Roentgenol. 2013; 200(6):1401–1408

[8] Haas BM, Kalra V, Geisel J, Raghu M, Durand M, Philpotts LE. Comparison of tomosynthesis plus digital mammography and digital mammography alone for breast cancer screening. Radiology. 2013; 269(3):694–700

[9] Friedewald SM, Rafferty EA, Rose SL, et al. Breast cancer screening using tomosynthesis in combination with digital mammography. JAMA. 2014; 311(24):2499–2507

[10] Sickles E, D'Orsi C, Bassett L, et al. ACR BI-RADS mammography. In: ACR BI-RADS Atlas, Breast Imaging Reporting and Data System. Reston, VA: American College of Radiology; 2013

[11] Kerlikowske K, Zhu W, Hubbard RA, et al. Breast Cancer Surveillance Consortium. Outcomes of screening mammography by frequency, breast density, and postmenopausal hormone therapy. JAMA Intern Med. 2013; 173 (9):807–816

[12] Carney PA, Miglioretti DL, Yankaskas BC, et al. Individual and combined effects of age, breast density, and hormone replacement therapy use on the accuracy of screening mammography. Ann Intern Med. 2003; 138(3):168–175

[13] Kerlikowske K, Hubbard RA, Miglioretti DL, et al. Breast Cancer Surveillance Consortium. Comparative effectiveness of digital versus film-screen mammography in community practice in the United States: a cohort study. Ann Intern Med. 2011; 155(8):493–502

[14] Pisano ED, Gatsonis C, Hendrick E, et al. Digital Mammographic Imaging Screening Trial (DMIST) Investigators Group. Diagnostic performance of digital versus film mammography for breast-cancer screening. N Engl J Med. 2005; 353 (17):1773–1783

[15] Boyd NF, Guo H, Martin LJ, et al. Mammographic density and the risk and detection of breast cancer. N Engl J Med. 2007; 356(3):227–236

[16] McCormack VA, dos Santos Silva I. Breast density and parenchymal patterns as markers of breast cancer risk: a meta-analysis. Cancer Epidemiol Biomarkers Prev. 2006; 15 (6):1159–1169

[17] Sickles EA. The use of breast imaging to screen women at high risk for cancer. Radiol Clin North Am. 2010; 48 (5):859–878

[18] Byrne C, Schairer C, Wolfe J, et al. Mammographic features and breast cancer risk: effects with time, age, and menopause status. J Natl Cancer Inst. 1995; 87(21):1622–1629

[19] Yaghjyan L, Colditz GA, Rosner B, Tamimi RM. Mammographic breast density and subsequent risk of breast cancer in postmenopausal women according to the time since the mammogram. Cancer Epidemiol Biomarkers Prev. 2013; 22 (6):1110–1117

[20] Price ER, Hargreaves J, Lipson JA, et al. The California breast density information group: a collaborative response to the issues of breast density, breast cancer risk, and breast density notification legislation. Radiology. 2013; 269(3):887–892

[21] Berg WA, Blume JD, Cormack JB, et al. ACRIN 6666 Investigators. Combined screening with ultrasound and mammography vs mammography alone in women at elevated risk of breast cancer. JAMA. 2008; 299(18):2151–2163

[22] Hooley RJ, Greenberg KL, Stackhouse RM, Geisel JL, Butler RS, Philpotts LE. Screening US in patients with mammographically dense breasts: initial experience with Connecticut Public Act 09–41. Radiology. 2012; 265(1):59–69

[23] Sprague BL, Stout NK, Schechter C, et al. Benefits, harms, and cost-effectiveness of supplemental ultrasonography screening for women with dense breasts. Ann Intern Med. 2015; 162(3):157–166

[24] Berg WA, Zhang Z, Lehrer D, et al. ACRIN 6666 Investigators. Detection of breast cancer with addition of annual screening ultrasound or a single screening MRI to mammography in women with elevated breast cancer risk. JAMA. 2012; 307 (13):1394–1404

[25] Kuhl CK, Schrading S, Strobel K, Schild HH, Hilgers RD, Bieling HB. Abbreviated breast magnetic resonance imaging (MRI): first postcontrast subtracted images and maximum-intensity projection-a novel approach to breast cancer screening with MRI. J Clin Oncol. 2014; 32(22):2304–2310

[26] Sung JS, Stamler S, Brooks J, et al. Breast cancers detected at screening MR imaging and mammography in patients at high risk: method of detection reflects tumor histopathologic results. Radiology. 2016; 280(3):716–722

[27] Lerner BH. "To see today with the eyes of tomorrow": a history of screening mammography. Can Bull Med Hist. 2003; 20(2):299–321

2 History of Magnetic Resonance Imaging in Breast Cancer Screening

Janice S. Sung and Elizabeth A. Morris

2.1 Introduction

Breast cancer is the most frequently diagnosed cancer in women in the United States, and the second leading cause of cancer death among women. In 2015, an estimated 231,840 new cases of invasive cancer were diagnosed, and approximately 40,290 women died of the disease.[1]

Mammography is the only imaging modality that has been validated by multiple randomized clinical trials and meta-analyses to reduce mortality from breast cancer.[2,3,4] Breast cancer mortality decreased by approximately 30% following implementation of mammographic screening programs, indicating that detecting cancers before they are clinically apparent reduces mortality. In addition, mammographic screening detects smaller, node-negative cancers, allowing patients to receive less aggressive surgical treatment and adjuvant therapy. Therefore, mammography is the primary modality for breast cancer screening in women at average risk for breast cancer. Earlier screening is recommended in some women who are at elevated risk for developing disease at a young age. For example, in women with a strong family history of breast cancer, screening mammography is recommended to begin 10 years earlier than the age at which the youngest first-degree family member was diagnosed.

Although effective in reducing mortality from breast cancer, mammography has its limitations, especially in young, high-risk women and in women with heterogeneously or extremely dense breasts. The false-negative rate of mammography may be as high as 20%, and increases to almost 50% in younger premenopausal average-risk women with dense breasts.[5] Breast cancers that occur in high-risk women, and especially cancers in women with a genetic predisposition, tend to be of a high nuclear grade, are more likely to be receptor negative, develop at an earlier age, and are more difficult to detect mammographically than sporadic breast cancers. The sensitivity of mammography in young high-risk women with dense breasts is reported to be as low as 38 to 50%.[6] Additionally, because breast cancers developing in women at genetic risk tend to be more aggressive, approximately half of mammographic screen-detected breast cancers in these women have nodal involvement at the time of diagnosis.[7,8,9]

Because of these shortcomings for mammography, other imaging modalities have been pursued as an adjunct screening modality in this population. Of these, the most widely accepted is contrast-enhanced breast magnetic resonance imaging (MRI). Advantages of MRI include its high sensitivity for invasive breast cancers. Unlike mammography, the sensitivity of MRI for cancer detection is not limited by breast density. This chapter will review the history of breast MRI and current recommendations of using breast MRI to screen asymptomatic women at high risk for breast cancer, and discuss the potential of an expanded role of breast MRI as a screening test with the advent of abbreviated breast MRI (AB-MR).

2.2 Importance of Early Detection: What Have We Learned from Mammography?

Multiple randomized controlled trials and observational and service studies in Europe and North America have demonstrated that breast cancer mortality decreases by approximately 30% once mammographic screening is instituted, suggesting that the early detection of breast cancers before they are clinically apparent reduces deaths due to breast cancer.[2,3,4,10] Meta-analyses have confirmed this reduction in breast cancer mortality begins 5 to 7 years after the institution of mammographic screening programs.[11]

In addition to reducing mortality, early detection through breast cancer screening also results in less invasive and aggressive therapy. The Swedish trials demonstrated that screening mammography detects small, node-negative breast cancers, allowing patients to receive less aggressive surgical as well as adjuvant therapy.[12] Therefore, early breast cancer detection through mammographic screening programs both reduces breast cancer morality and improves treatment options.

Although mammography is an effective screening test, the limitations of mammography discussed earlier, particularly in high-risk women and in women with dense breasts, have led to interest in other modalities to supplement mammographic screening. Any alternative or supplemental screening test has been measured by its ability to detect small node-negative breast cancers.

2.3 Early Research on Breast MRI

Research in the use of breast MRI began in the 1980s in the United States and Germany. Breast MRI was initially performed in the early 1980s using a body coil, but dedicated breast coils were soon developed by the mid-1980s.[13,14,15] In 1986, Heywang et al demonstrated that cancers on breast MRIs performed following gadolinium administration demonstrated increased enhancement relative to the normal breast parenchyma, findings confirmed on subsequent studies (▶ Fig. 2.1).[16,17] Most breast cancers demonstrate early enhancement (rapid wash), while the normal breast parenchyma progressively enhances with time. Therefore, neoplasms are most discernible in the early postcontrast phase, approximately 60 to 120 seconds after contrast injection.

During the 1990s, efforts were directed at improving image acquisition and interpretation. Much debate centered on whether the emphasis should be on enhancement kinetics or lesion morphology. Was it more important to detect a washout kinetic pattern indicating possible angiogenesis associated with invasive cancer or obtain detailed information on morphology to distinguish a benign from malignant lesion? High temporal resolution implies rapid image acquisition in order to maximize information on lesion kinetics, while high spatial resolution imaging obtains thin slices in order to maximize information on lesion morphology. High spatial resolution images (slice thickness ≤3 mm and <1 mm in plane resolution) are necessary to both detect small lesions and assess their morphology (▶ Fig. 2.2). Therefore, improving spatial resolution and increasing temporal resolution represent competing interests. Any increase in spatial resolution requires an increase in acquisition time.

Reducing temporal resolution decreases sampling rate, which may lead to a loss in the ability to detect changes in signal intensity. Kuhl et al examined the trade-off between spatial and temporal resolution. Although there is a loss of kinetic

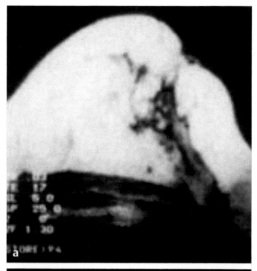
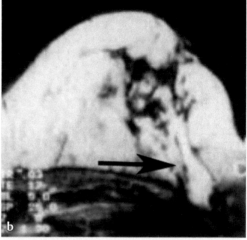

Fig. 2.1 Early breast magnetic resonance imaging (MRI). Axial images of an enhancing breast cancer (*black arrow*) on an early breast MRI performed in 1989 (**a**) before and (**b**) after intravenous gadolinium injection. (Adapted with permission from Kaiser and Zeitler[17].)

information when reducing temporal resolution and increasing spatial resolution, kinetic information is usually preserved with acquisition times of 2 minutes or less due to the broad overlap of enhancement rates between benign and malignant lesions, with the benefit of gaining improved morphological information.[18] Current full breast MRI protocols are performed on either 1.5- or 3-T magnets and provide both high spatial resolution (≤3 mm slices with ≤1 mm in-plane spatial resolution) and high temporal resolution (acquisition time within ≤2 min).

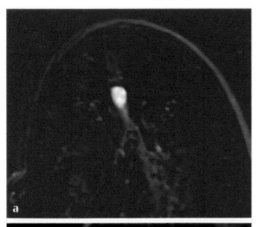

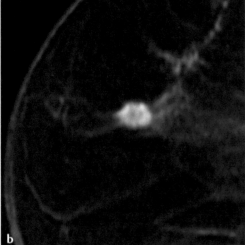

Fig. 2.2 Importance of high spatial resolution. (a) Axial subtracted image from a low spatial resolution magnetic resonance imaging (MRI) demonstrates what appears to be a circumscribed homogeneously enhancing mass with nonenhancing internal septations, suggestive of a fibroadenoma. (b) The same lesion imaged at high resolution demonstrates spiculated, irregular rim enhancing mass. Biopsy yielded invasive ductal carcinoma.

2.4 MRI for High-Risk Screening

Initial studies reported a very high sensitivity of breast MRI for invasive cancers, spurring interest in the possibility of using MRI as a supplemental screening modality.[17,19,20] Kuhl et al published the first study on using breast MRI to screen women at high risk for breast cancer.[21] This study included 192 women with a suspected or known carrier of a breast cancer susceptibility gene. In that study, six

of the nine cancers diagnosed were seen only on MRI and occult on both mammography and ultrasound, demonstrating a significantly higher accuracy of breast MRI compared to conventional imaging when used to screen high-risk women.

In 2004, Kriege et al published their results from the Netherlands comparing the sensitivity of MRI to mammography and clinical breast exam in one of the largest screening MRI trials, which included 1,909 women. In this study, the sensitivity of MRI was 79.5% compared to 17.9% for clinical breast exam and 33% for mammography.[22] Multiple subsequent studies confirmed the substantially higher sensitivity of breast MRI for invasive cancers compared to both mammography and ultrasound, resulting in current recommendations of annual screening MRI as an adjunct to annual mammography in women at high risk for breast cancer (▶ Fig. 2.3; ▶ Table 2.1).[22,23,24,25,26,27,28] Supplemental screening with breast MRI is recommended by the American Cancer Society (ACS), the National Comprehensive Cancer Network (NCCN), and joint recommendations from the Society of Breast Imaging (SBI) and the American College of Radiology (ACR) for patients with a known *BRCA1* or *BRCA2* mutation and for their untested first-degree relatives, for women with a lifetime risk of 20 to 25% or greater, and for women with a history of chest irradiation.[29,30] Annual screening with MRI and mammography is also recommended for women with Li–Fraumeni syndrome, Cowden syndrome, or Bannayan–Riley–Ruvalcaba syndrome.

2.4.1 Hereditary/Familial Risk of Breast Cancer

Genetic abnormalities account for 5 to 10% of all cases of breast cancer.[31] The most well-known are mutations involving the *BRCA1* and *BRCA2* genes, identified in the 1990s.[32] The prevalence of a BRCA mutation is approximately 1/500 to 1/1,000 in the general population and 1/50 in women with a Jewish ancestry. The estimated risk for breast cancer by the age of 70 ranges from 46 to 87% with a *BRCA1* mutation and 37 to 84% with a *BRCA2* mutation.[33] The BRCA1 gene, located on chromosome 17, is a tumor suppressor gene. The *BRCA1* gene is thought to be responsible for the breast/ovarian syndrome, and accounts for 50% of familial breast cancers and 5 to 8% of all breast cancers. The relative risk associated with a *BRCA1* mutation declines with advancing age. The *BRCA2* gene is located on chromosome 13 and accounts for

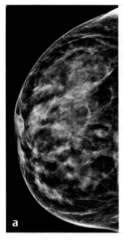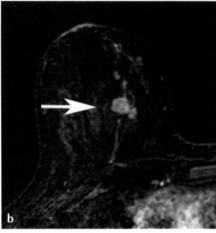

Fig. 2.3 Mammographically occult breast cancer. (**a**) Right craniocaudal (CC) view from a digital breast tomosynthesis study demonstrates no abnormality. (**b**) Axial subtracted image demonstrates an irregular heterogeneously enhancing mass (*white arrow*) in the medial right breast. Biopsy yielded invasive ductal carcinoma.

Table 2.1 Summary of selected prospective trials comparing screening with mammography, US, and MRI in women at high risk for breast cancer

Author (year)	CA/No. of women (%)	Sensitivity			Specificity		
		MG (%)	US (%)	MR (%)	MG (%)	US (%)	MR (%)
Kriege et al (2004)[22]	50/1,909 (3)	40	–	71	95	–	90
Warner et al (2004)[28]	22/236 (9)	36	33	77	100	96	95
Kuhl et al (2005)[23]	43/529 (8)	33	40	91	97	91	97
Leach et al (2005)[24]	35/649 (5)	40	–	77	93	–	81
Hagen et al (2007)[25]	25/491 (5)	50	–	86	–	–	–
Rijnsburger et al (2010)[26]	97/2,157 (4)	41	–	71	95	–	90
Sardanelli et al (2011)[27]	52/501 (10)	50	52	91	99	98	97

Abbreviations: CA, cancer; MG, mammography; MRI, magnetic resonance imaging; US, ultrasound.

approximately 35% of familial breast cancers. *BRCA2* carriers are at risk for developing other cancers, including prostate, bladder, pancreatic, and Hodgkin's disease. Mutations in other genes, such as the *TP53* and *PTEN* genes among others, are also known to confer a high risk for breast cancer but are much less common.[34]

There has been increasing recognition of the role of tumor biology in *BRCA1* and *BRCA2* mutation carriers. *BRCA1*-related breast cancers differ from sporadic cancers in that they are often of higher histological grade, show lymphocytic infiltration, and are more likely to be aneuploid and triple negative (estrogen, progesterone, and human epidermal growth factor 2 receptor negative).[35,36] The interval cancer rate, that is, cancers detected in between annual screening, is also known to be high in *BRCA* mutation carriers, due to the rapid tumor growth rate in these women.[9] Studies have also shown that in *BRCA1* or *BRCA2* mutation carriers, the tumor growth rate is double that of nonmutation carriers and is highest in women who develop breast cancer at the youngest ages.[37]

Despite the widespread evidence that mammographic screening improves mortality in the general population, there is little evidence that mammographic screening reduces cancer mortality in high-risk mutation carriers. Evans et al compared survival rates in women with a likely or known *BRCA1*, *BRCA2*, or *TP53* mutation that were not being screened for breast cancer, screened with mammography alone, or screened with a combination of mammography and MR.[38] There was a significant survival benefit for those women undergoing surveillance compared to those not screened, and a borderline significant advantage in survival between those screened with a combination of mammography and MRI compared to those screened with mammography alone.

Multiple retrospective and prospective studies have demonstrated the limitations of mammography in high-risk patients, especially in those with a *BRCA* mutation. The sensitivity of mammography in young, high-risk women with dense breast tissue is consistently reported to be less than 50%. In addition, of the cancers detected, 40 to 78% of the invasive cancers are greater than 1 cm in diameter and axillary nodes are involved in 20 to 56%.[7,8,9] Explanations for the low sensitivity of mammography in these studies may include the higher breast density in younger women, a higher likelihood of rapidly growing tumors, and the more benign appearance of many *BRCA1* cancers, making them more difficult to detect.[6]

Only 1 to 2% of women have a family history suggestive of an autosomal dominant gene mutation. Although the majority of women in the general population have at least one relative with a history of breast cancer, this does not confer an increased risk because that cancer was sporadic or confers a low increase in risk due to a low penetrance gene. Features that suggest that the breast cancer may be due to a high penetrance gene include two or more close relatives with breast or ovarian cancer, breast cancer occurring before age 50 in a close relative, a family history of both breast and ovarian cancer, one or more relatives with two cancers (breast and ovarian cancer or two independent breast cancers), and male relatives with breast cancer.

Supplemental screening with breast MRI is also recommended for women with a lifetime breast cancer risk of greater than 20 to 25%. Multiple models are available to assign risk, including Gail, Claus, Tyrer-Cuzick, Breast and Ovarian Analysis of

Disease Incidence and Carrier Estimation Algorithm (BOADICEA), and BRCAPRO models.[39,40,41,42,43] Each of these risk assessment models incorporates different risk factors to calculate the breast cancer risk. The Gail model does not factor in a family history other than a first-degree relative and is specifically not recommended to be used to determine whether supplemental screening with MRI is indicated.[44] The Tyrer-Cuzick model includes both family history and a history of high-risk lesions such as lobular carcinoma in situ (LCIS) and atypical ductal hyperplasia (ADH), which are not included in the other risk assessment models.[45] Because each model incorporates different risk factors, the calculated lifetime risk may vary widely depending on the model used. For example, the lifetime risk of a 35-year-old woman with a mother diagnosed with breast cancer at the age of 51 and a maternal aunt diagnosed with breast cancer at the age of 60 would have a BRACAPRO lifetime risk of 13%, a Claus risk of 18%, and a Tyrer-Cuzick risk of 23%.[46]

As discussed earlier, starting from the mid-1990s, multiple prospective studies were performed to evaluate the utility of MRI as an adjunctive screening tool in women with a known or likely genetic mutation predisposing them to breast cancer.[22,23,24,28,47,48,49,50] The risk factors of the women included in these studies vary widely, with some studies including only women with a known or high suspicion for a *BRCA* mutation and others including women with a wide range of risk factors including a strong family history or personal history of breast cancer or prior biopsy demonstrating LCIS or ADH. Despite these differences, the sensitivity of breast MRI in all these studies was significantly higher than that of mammography, with a sensitivity of approximately 90%. In these trials, the sensitivity of MRI ranged from 71 to 100%, compared to 13 to 59% for mammography. When data from 11 studies were combined in a meta-analysis, it was found that there was a sensitivity of 77% for MRI alone, 94% for a combination of MRI and mammography, and 39% for mammography alone.[51] Therefore, the highest sensitivity was achieved using a combination of mammography and MRI. The addition of ultrasound has not been shown to improve cancer detection rates beyond that achieved with MRI and mammography.[52]

The prevalence of mammographically occult breast cancer in the first round of screening MRI is extremely high at between 1.1 and 10%, which is about 10 times the expected rate in the general population.[53] In studies where more than one round of MRI screening was performed, the incidence was found to be between 0.6 and 4%, indicating a continued benefit to MRI screening in this population after the first screening round. While some of these studies include women with a "strong family history" of breast cancer or other risk factors, it is not surprising that the highest cancer detection rates were reported in those studies evaluating patients with *BRCA1* and *BRCA2* mutations.

Based on these trials, the recommended screening algorithm for women at high risk for hereditary breast cancer is a combination of mammography and MRI. A recent modeling study reported that the most efficacious screening strategy for *BRCA* mutation carriers in terms of increased life expectancy weighed against false positives was to start screening with MRI annually at age 25 and to add annual mammography at age 30, staggering the two examinations at 6-month intervals.[54] Since breast cancer rarely develops before age 25 years in these women, screening should not commence earlier than this age.

2.4.2 History of Chest Irradiation

Patients with a history of pediatric or young adult cancers are at increased risk of breast cancer if treatment of their childhood cancer included mediastinal/chest irradiation. The risk of subsequent development of breast cancer is highest in women treated between the ages of 10 and 30 years, due to the sensitivity of breast tissue to radiation during this period.[55,56] The cumulative risk increases with the radiation dose delivered, volume of the radiation field, and time interval since completion of the radiation therapy.[57]

Breast cancer is the leading cause of death in women who are long-term survivors of Hodgkin's lymphoma.[55,56,58,59,60,61,62] The incidence of breast cancer is similar to that of women with a *BRCA* mutation. By the age of 40 to 45 years, approximately 13% to 20% of women treated with moderate- to high-dose chest irradiation for a pediatric cancer will be diagnosed with breast cancer.[58,60,63]

Currently, annual screening mammography and MRI are recommended beginning 8 years following completion of chest irradiation but not before the age of 25 years.[63,64] However, approximately 50 to 60% of mammograms in women between the ages of 25 to 55 years who were treated with chest irradiation have moderate to very dense breast tissue, limiting the sensitivity of mammography.[65,66] Therefore, the ACS, the ACR, the SBI, and the

Children's Oncology Group recommend annual screening MRI as an adjunct to mammography in women with a history of chest irradiation.[29,67] Two retrospective studies have evaluated the utility of screening breast MRI in detecting mammographically occult breast cancers in women with a history of chest irradiation. Sung et al reported a 4.4% incremental cancer detection rate of screening breast MRI over mammography.[68] The mammographically occult, MRI-detected cancers were early-stage, T1 invasive cancers. Freitas et al similarly reported a 4.1% added cancer detection rate using MRI to screen patients with a history of chest radiation.[69]

The increased incidence of breast cancer in this population underscores the importance of breast cancer screening. However, one study surveying women treated with chest irradiation between the ages of 25 and 50 in the United States and Canada found that almost 50% of women between the ages of 25 and 39 had never had a mammogram, and less than 2% had undergone a screening breast MRI.[64]

2.5 Intermediate-Risk Women

Women at intermediate risk for breast cancer are those with a 15 to 20% lifetime risk, and may include women with a history of LCIS, ADH, or a personal history of breast cancer. The ACS guidelines state that there is insufficient evidence to recommend for or against MRI screening; the NCCN and SBI/ACR guidelines state that MRI should be considered in these patients.

2.5.1 History of Lobular Carcinoma In Situ

A biopsy-proven diagnosis of LCIS is associated with a 7 to 12 increased relative risk of breast cancer.[70,71] The true incidence of LCIS is unknown, as LCIS is rarely mammographically visible, and is usually an incidental histologic finding in tissue samples obtained for another lesion either from percutaneous biopsy or in a surgical specimen performed for other reasons. LCIS is currently considered to be a risk indicator for developing subsequent breast cancer in either breast or a nonobligate precursor for invasive lobular carcinoma.[70,72,73] The time interval from the initial diagnosis of LCIS to the development of a subsequent cancer has been reported to be greater than 15 years in more than 50% of cases.[71,74]

A few retrospective single institution retrospective studies have evaluated the utility of screening MRI in this population. Port et al included women with a history of either atypical hyperplasia or LCIS and reported MRI-detected malignancies in 4% of patients with LCIS and in no patients with atypical hyperplasia.[75] Sung et al also reported an additional cancer detection rate of 4.5% of screening breast MRI over mammography in women with LCIS only, and found that the majority of mammographically occult cancers detected on screening MRI were early T1 invasive cancers.[76] Similarly, Friedlander et al reported that screening MRI-detected malignancy in 3.8% of patients with LCIS, with a median size of 0.8 cm for MRI-detected cancers.[77]

2.5.2 Personal History of Breast Cancer

Women with a personal history of breast cancer may also fall within the 15 to 20% lifetime intermediate breast cancer risk category depending on their age at cancer diagnosis and the presence of other risk factors. Tumor recurrence rates after breast conservation therapy have historically been estimated at approximately 1 to 2% per year.[78] However, recurrence rates at 10 years are now less than 10% due to improvements in chemotherapy and hormonal therapy.

Due to normal posttreatment-related changes such as architectural distortion and increased density at the lumpectomy site, only about 24 to 45% are mammographically detected.[79,80] However, early detection of treatment failures improves relative survival by 27 to 47%.[81] Conversely, recurrent disease that is either large or node positive indicates a poorer prognosis.

Several retrospective studies have reported a higher sensitivity with MRI in detecting subclinical recurrent disease. Brennan et al reported that breast cancer was detected on MRI in 12% of women with a personal history of breast cancer.[80] All of the cancers seen on MRI were minimal cancers, defined as either ductal carcinoma in situ or node-negative breast cancers < 1 cm in size. Gweon et al found an additional 18.1 cancers per 1,000 women with a personal breast cancer history on MRI who had a negative mammogram and ultrasound.[82] The invasive cancers detected on MRI were all node negative, with a median size of 0.8 cm. The positive predictive value (PPV) of biopsy was 43.5%. Yang et al also found that women with mammographically occult breast cancer were more likely to develop breast recurrences that also were mammographically occult, suggesting that supplemental imaging modalities such as MRI may be particularly useful in this subgroup of women.[83] Recently, Lehman et al reported that the diagnostic performance of screening MRI is superior for women with a personal history of breast cancer compared with women with a genetic or family history of cancer.[84]

2.6 Survival Benefit from Screening MR

Although it is clear that MRI is the most sensitive modality for breast cancer detection, no randomized or prospective clinical trial has demonstrated a mortality reduction due to supplemental screening with breast MRI. Currently, tumor size and nodal status are used as surrogate markers of mortality, since tumor stage at the time of diagnosis remains the most important determinant of outcome. The 5-year relative survival of breast cancer localized to the breast at the time of diagnosis is 98.6%, compared to 83.8% with regional disease, and 23.3% with distant metastases.[85] Several studies have shown that cancers detected on screening breast MRI are significantly smaller and have lower rates of nodal involvement compared to those detected on mammography.[22,50,86] Therefore, it is likely that early detection with screening breast MRI also translates into a mortality reduction.

2.7 Future of Breast MRI Screening

The use of MRI for breast cancer screening has remained largely unchanged for the past 10 years primarily due to the time required to perform the study and high cost compared to mammography. This includes the cost of not only screening MRI but also any follow-up imaging or biopsies recommended from that screening MRI. In almost all of the early high-risk screening trials, the specificity of MRI was lower than that of mammography. However, with increased experience, the current 6-month follow-up recommendation rates and PPV3 of biopsy for MRI are comparable to that of mammography.

The landscape of breast cancer screening for women at average to intermediate risk has changed in recent years due to the passage of breast density legislation. Twenty-four states have passed breast density legislation, which requires that women be informed if they have mammographically hetero-geneously dense or extremely dense breasts and that supplemental breast cancer screening be considered. These laws impact a very large number of women; more than 50% of women younger than 50 years and at least 33% of women older than 50 have dense breasts.[87] Due to its wide availability, ultrasound has become the primary supplemental imaging modality to screen women with dense breasts that are at average or intermediate risk for breast cancer. Multiple studies have consistently shown that screening breast ultrasound will detect an additional 2 to 4 mammographically occult cancers per 1,000 women screened.[88,89,90] Therefore, the current standard screening practice for women with dense breasts in many states is annual mammography supplemented by whole breast screening ultrasound. However, screening breast ultrasound has a number of limitations including time, cost, and a low positive predictive value of biopsy (PPV3) of approximately 8%, leading to a significant number of unnecessary biopsies and a much higher rate of recommendation for short-term interval follow-up.[88,89] The combination of mammography and supplemental screening breast ultrasound represents a burden on health care costs. Sprague et al[91] estimated the cost per quality-adjusted life-year (QALY) gained by screening mammogram with supplemental ultrasound was $320,000.

Due to the low PPV3 of biopsy, time required to perform, and cost associated with screening breast ultrasound and the biopsies and follow-up studies generated from the study, alternative supplemental screening tests have been investigated to screen women with dense breasts. One alternative is AB-MR, where the scan time is reduced to less than 10 minutes in order to reduce the time and cost of the MRI so that it is comparable to the current standard combination of mammography and screening breast ultrasound. Kuhl et al prospectively evaluated an AB-MR protocol consisting of one T1-weighted precontrast and one postcontrast series and their derived images prior to evaluating the full diagnostic protocoling for 606 screening breast MRIs.[92] The diagnostic accuracy of the abbreviated protocol was equivalent to the full diagnostic protocol, yielding an incremental cancer detection rate of 18.2 per 1,000. Using the abbreviated protocol, the acquisition time was reduced to 3 minutes. Another study retrospectively evaluated

images of an AB-MR protocol in 100 patients with known cancer, and found a sensitivity of 96% using only the first postcontrast and subtraction images.[93] With AB-MR, the fast image acquisition time and interpretation time could markedly reduce the costs of screening breast MRI and allow for increased availability to a broader population. AB-MR may become the best supplemental screening tests for average- and intermediate-risk women with dense breasts, replacing the current standard but suboptimal combination of mammography and screening breast ultrasound.

2.8 Conclusion

Breast MRI was first investigated in the 1980s and has become the mainstay for supplemental screening of high-risk women due to its high sensitivity for breast cancer detection compared to conventional imaging. Despite its high sensitivity, breast MRI has been restricted to screening of high-risk women primarily due to its high cost. Due to the passage of breast density legislation in 24 states, new modalities are being investigated for supplemental breast cancer screening in women with dense breasts. The advent of AB-MR, which reduces the cost of MRI to that comparable to conventional imaging techniques, represents a promising new tool and may be the optimal supplemental screening test for average- and intermediate-risk women with dense breasts.

References

[1] American Cancer Society. Cancer Facts & Figures 2015. Atlanta, CA: American Cancer Society; 2015

[2] Smith RA, Duffy SW, Gabe R, Tabar L, Yen AM, Chen TH. The randomized trials of breast cancer screening: what have we learned? Radiol Clin North Am. 2004; 42(5):793–806, v

[3] Shapiro S, Strax P, Venet L. Periodic breast cancer screening in reducing mortality from breast cancer. JAMA. 1971; 215 (11):1777–1785

[4] Tabár L, Vitak B, Chen TH, et al. Swedish two-county trial: impact of mammographic screening on breast cancer mortality during 3 decades. Radiology. 2011; 260(3):658–663

[5] Kolb TM, Lichy J, Newhouse JH. Comparison of the performance of screening mammography, physical examination, and breast US and evaluation of factors that influence them: an analysis of 27,825 patient evaluations. Radiology. 2002; 225 (1):165–175

[6] Tilanus-Linthorst M, Verhoog L, Obdeijn IM, et al. A BRCA1/2 mutation, high breast density and prominent pushing margins of a tumor independently contribute to a frequent false-negative mammography. Int J Cancer. 2002; 102(1):91–95

[7] Brekelmans CT, Seynaeve C, Bartels CC, et al. Rotterdam Committee for Medical and Genetic Counseling. Effectiveness of breast cancer surveillance in BRCA1/2 gene mutation carriers

and women with high familial risk. J Clin Oncol. 2001; 19 (4):924–930

[8] Scheuer L, Kauff N, Robson M, et al. Outcome of preventive surgery and screening for breast and ovarian cancer in BRCA mutation carriers. J Clin Oncol. 2002; 20(5):1260–1268

[9] Komenaka IK, Ditkoff BA, Joseph KA, et al. The development of interval breast malignancies in patients with BRCA mutations. Cancer. 2004; 100(10):2079–2083

[10] Nickson C, Mason KE, English DR, Kavanagh AM. Mammographic screening and breast cancer mortality: a case-control study and meta-analysis. Cancer Epidemiol Biomarkers Prev. 2012; 21(9):1479–1488

[11] Kerlikowske K, Grady D, Rubin SM, Sandrock C, Ernster VL. Efficacy of screening mammography. A meta-analysis. JAMA. 1995; 273(2):149–154

[12] Tabár L, Vitak B, Chen HH, et al. The Swedish Two-County Trial twenty years later. Updated mortality results and new insights from long-term follow-up. Radiol Clin North Am. 2000; 38(4):625–651

[13] Ross RJ, Thompson JS, Kim K, Bailey RA. Nuclear magnetic resonance imaging and evaluation of human breast tissue: preliminary clinical trials. Radiology. 1982; 143(1):195–205

[14] El Yousef SJ, Duchesneau RH, Alfidi RJ, Haaga JR, Bryan PJ, LiPuma JP. Magnetic resonance imaging of the breast. Work in progress. Radiology. 1984; 150(3):761–766

[15] Stelling CB, Wang PC, Lieber A, Mattingly SS, Griffen WO, Powell DE. Prototype coil for magnetic resonance imaging of the female breast. Work in progress. Radiology. 1985; 154 (2):457–462

[16] Heywang SH, Hahn D, Schmidt H, et al. MR imaging of the breast using gadolinium-DTPA. J Comput Assist Tomogr. 1986; 10(2):199–204

[17] Kaiser WA, Zeitler E. MR imaging of the breast: fast imaging sequences with and without Gd-DTPA. Preliminary observations. Radiology. 1989; 170(3, Pt 1):681–686

[18] Kuhl CK, Schild HH, Morakkabati N. Dynamic bilateral contrast-enhanced MR imaging of the breast: trade-off between spatial and temporal resolution. Radiology. 2005; 236 (3):789–800

[19] Harms SE, Flamig DP, Hesley KL, et al. MR imaging of the breast with rotating delivery of excitation off resonance: clinical experience with pathologic correlation. Radiology. 1993; 187(2):493–501

[20] Heywang SH, Wolf A, Pruss E, Hilbertz T, Eiermann W, Permanetter W. MR imaging of the breast with Gd-DTPA: use and limitations. Radiology. 1989; 171(1):95–103

[21] Kuhl CK, Schmutzler RK, Leutner CC, et al. Breast MR imaging screening in 192 women proved or suspected to be carriers of a breast cancer susceptibility gene: preliminary results. Radiology. 2000; 215(1):267–279

[22] Kriege M, Brekelmans CT, Boetes C, et al. Magnetic Resonance Imaging Screening Study Group. Efficacy of MRI and mammography for breast-cancer screening in women with a familial or genetic predisposition. N Engl J Med. 2004; 351 (5):427–437

[23] Kuhl CK, Schrading S, Leutner CC, et al. Mammography, breast ultrasound, and magnetic resonance imaging for surveillance of women at high familial risk for breast cancer. J Clin Oncol. 2005; 23(33):8469–8476

[24] Leach MO, Boggis CR, Dixon AK, et al. MARIBS study group. Screening with magnetic resonance imaging and mammography of a UK population at high familial risk of breast cancer: a prospective multicentre cohort study (MARIBS). Lancet. 2005; 365(9473):1769–1778

[25] Hagen AI, Kvistad KA, Maehle L, et al. Sensitivity of MRI versus conventional screening in the diagnosis of BRCA-

associated breast cancer in a national prospective series. Breast. 2007; 16(4):367–374

[26] Rijnsburger AJ, Obdeijn IM, Kaas R, et al. BRCA1-associated breast cancers present differently from BRCA2-associated and familial cases: long-term follow-up of the Dutch MRISC Screening Study. J Clin Oncol. 2010; 28(36):5265–5273

[27] Sardanelli F, Podo F, Santoro F, et al. High Breast Cancer Risk Italian 1 (HIBCRIT-1) Study. Multicenter surveillance of women at high genetic breast cancer risk using mammography, ultrasonography, and contrast-enhanced magnetic resonance imaging (the high breast cancer risk Italian 1 study): final results. Invest Radiol. 2011; 46(2):94–105

[28] Warner E, Plewes DB, Hill KA, et al. Surveillance of BRCA1 and BRCA2 mutation carriers with magnetic resonance imaging, ultrasound, mammography, and clinical breast examination. JAMA. 2004; 292(11):1317–1325

[29] Saslow D, Boetes C, Burke W, et al. American Cancer Society Breast Cancer Advisory Group. American Cancer Society guidelines for breast screening with MRI as an adjunct to mammography. CA Cancer J Clin. 2007; 57(2):75–89

[30] Bevers TB, Anderson BO, Bonaccio E, et al. National Comprehensive Cancer Network. NCCN clinical practice guidelines in oncology: breast cancer screening and diagnosis. J Natl Compr Canc Netw. 2009; 7(10):1060–1096

[31] Garber JE, Offit K. Hereditary cancer predisposition syndromes. J Clin Oncol. 2005; 23(2):276–292

[32] Narod SA, Foulkes WD. BRCA1 and BRCA2: 1994 and beyond. Nat Rev Cancer. 2004; 4(9):665–676

[33] Sickles EA. The use of breast imaging to screen women at high risk for cancer. Radiol Clin North Am. 2010; 48 (5):859–878

[34] Foulkes WD. Inherited susceptibility to common cancers. N Engl J Med. 2008; 359(20):2143–2153

[35] Rakha EA, Reis-Filho JS, Ellis IO. Basal-like breast cancer: a critical review. J Clin Oncol. 2008; 26(15):2568–2581

[36] Chappuis PO, Nethercot V, Foulkes WD. Clinico-pathological characteristics of BRCA1- and BRCA2-related breast cancer. Semin Surg Oncol. 2000; 18(4):287–295

[37] Tilanus-Linthorst MM, Obdeijn IM, Hop WC, et al. BRCA1 mutation and young age predict fast breast cancer growth in the Dutch, United Kingdom, and Canadian magnetic resonance imaging screening trials. Clin Cancer Res. 2007; 13 (24):7357–7362

[38] Evans DG, Kesavan N, Lim Y, et al. MARIBS Group. MRI breast screening in high-risk women: cancer detection and survival analysis. Breast Cancer Res Treat. 2014; 145(3):663–672

[39] Gail MH, Brinton LA, Byar DP, et al. Projecting individualized probabilities of developing breast cancer for white females who are being examined annually. J Natl Cancer Inst. 1989; 81(24):1879–1886

[40] Claus EB, Risch N, Thompson WD. Autosomal dominant inheritance of early-onset breast cancer. Implications for risk prediction. Cancer. 1994; 73(3):643–651

[41] Tyrer J, Duffy SW, Cuzick J. A breast cancer prediction model incorporating familial and personal risk factors. Stat Med. 2004; 23(7):1111–1130

[42] Berry DA, Iversen ES, Jr, Gudbjartsson DF, et al. BRCAPRO validation, sensitivity of genetic testing of BRCA1/BRCA2, and prevalence of other breast cancer susceptibility genes. J Clin Oncol. 2002; 20(11):2701–2712

[43] Antoniou AC, Cunningham AP, Peto J, et al. The BOADICEA model of genetic susceptibility to breast and ovarian cancers: updates and extensions. Br J Cancer. 2008; 98(8):1457–1466

[44] Berg WA. Tailored supplemental screening for breast cancer: what now and what next? AJR Am J Roentgenol. 2009; 192 (2):390–399

[45] Evans DG, Howell A. Breast cancer risk-assessment models. Breast Cancer Res. 2007; 9(5):213

[46] Jochelson MS, Morris EA. An imaging approach to high-risk screening for breast cancer. Semin Roentgenol. 2011; 46 (1):68–75

[47] Hartman AR, Daniel BL, Kurian AW, et al. Breast magnetic resonance image screening and ductal lavage in women at high genetic risk for breast carcinoma. Cancer. 2004; 100(3):479–489

[48] Lehman CD, Isaacs C, Schnall MD, et al. Cancer yield of mammography, MR, and US in high-risk women: prospective multi-institution breast cancer screening study. Radiology. 2007; 244(2):381–388

[49] Sardanelli F, Podo F, D'Agnolo G, et al. High Breast Cancer Risk Italian Trial. Multicenter comparative multimodality surveillance of women at genetic-familial high risk for breast cancer (HIBCRIT study): interim results. Radiology. 2007; 242 (3):698–715

[50] Lehman CD, Blume JD, Weatherall P, et al. International Breast MRI Consortium Working Group. Screening women at high risk for breast cancer with mammography and magnetic resonance imaging. Cancer. 2005; 103(9):1898–1905

[51] Warner E, Messersmith H, Causer P, Eisen A, Shumak R, Plewes D. Systematic review: using magnetic resonance imaging to screen women at high risk for breast cancer. Ann Intern Med. 2008; 148(9):671–679

[52] Kuhl C, Weigel S, Schrading S, et al. Prospective multicenter cohort study to refine management recommendations for women at elevated familial risk of breast cancer: the EVA trial. J Clin Oncol. 2010; 28(9):1450–1457

[53] Warner E. Impact of MRI surveillance and breast cancer detection in young women with BRCA mutations. Ann Oncol. 2011; 22 Suppl 1:i44–i49

[54] Lowry KP, Lee JM, Kong CY, et al. Annual screening strategies in BRCA1 and BRCA2 gene mutation carriers: a comparative effectiveness analysis. Cancer. 2012; 118(8):2021–2030

[55] Hancock SL, Tucker MA, Hoppe RT. Breast cancer after treatment of Hodgkin's disease. J Natl Cancer Inst. 1993; 85 (1):25–31

[56] Travis LB, Hill DA, Dores GM, et al. Breast cancer following radiotherapy and chemotherapy among young women with Hodgkin disease. JAMA. 2003; 290(4):465–475

[57] Travis LB, Hill D, Dores GM, et al. Cumulative absolute breast cancer risk for young women treated for Hodgkin lymphoma. J Natl Cancer Inst. 2005; 97(19):1428–1437

[58] Bhatia S, Yasui Y, Robison LL, et al. Late Effects Study Group. High risk of subsequent neoplasms continues with extended follow-up of childhood Hodgkin's disease: report from the Late Effects Study Group. J Clin Oncol. 2003; 21(23):4386–4394

[59] Guibout C, Adjadj E, Rubino C, et al. Malignant breast tumors after radiotherapy for a first cancer during childhood. J Clin Oncol. 2005; 23(1):197–204

[60] Kenney LB, Yasui Y, Inskip PD, et al. Breast cancer after childhood cancer: a report from the Childhood Cancer Survivor Study. Ann Intern Med. 2004; 141(8):590–597

[61] Bhatia S, Robison LL, Oberlin O, et al. Breast cancer and other second neoplasms after childhood Hodgkin's disease. N Engl J Med. 1996; 334(12):745–751

[62] Mertens AC, Liu Q, Neglia JP, et al. Cause-specific late mortality among 5-year survivors of childhood cancer: the Childhood Cancer Survivor Study. J Natl Cancer Inst. 2008; 100 (19):1368–1379

[63] Henderson TO, Amsterdam A, Bhatia S, et al. Systematic review: surveillance for breast cancer in women treated with chest radiation for childhood, adolescent, or young adult cancer. Ann Intern Med. 2010; 152(7):444–455, W144–W154

[64] Oeffinger KC, Ford JS, Moskowitz CS, et al. Breast cancer surveillance practices among women previously treated with chest radiation for a childhood cancer. JAMA. 2009; 301 (4):404–414

[65] Kwong A, Hancock SL, Bloom JR, et al. Mammographic screening in women at increased risk of breast cancer after treatment of Hodgkin's disease. Breast J. 2008; 14(1):39–48

[66] Lee L, Pintilie M, Hodgson DC, Goss PE, Crump M. Screening mammography for young women treated with supradiaphragmatic radiation for Hodgkin's lymphoma. Ann Oncol. 2008; 19(1):62–67

[67] Lee CH, Dershaw DD, Kopans D, et al. Breast cancer screening with imaging: recommendations from the Society of Breast Imaging and the ACR on the use of mammography, breast MRI, breast ultrasound, and other technologies for the detection of clinically occult breast cancer. J Am Coll Radiol. 2010; 7(1):18–27

[68] Sung JS, Lee CH, Morris EA, Oeffinger KC, Dershaw DD. Screening breast MR imaging in women with a history of chest irradiation. Radiology. 2011; 259(1):65–71

[69] Freitas V, Scaranelo A, Menezes R, Kulkarni S, Hodgson D, Crystal P. Added cancer yield of breast magnetic resonance imaging screening in women with a prior history of chest radiation therapy. Cancer. 2013; 119(3):495–503

[70] Simpson PT, Gale T, Fulford LG, Reis-Filho JS, Lakhani SR. The diagnosis and management of pre-invasive breast disease: pathology of atypical lobular hyperplasia and lobular carcinoma in situ. Breast Cancer Res. 2003; 5(5):258–262

[71] Arpino G, Laucirica R, Elledge RM. Premalignant and in situ breast disease: biology and clinical implications. Ann Intern Med. 2005; 143(6):446–457

[72] Li CI, Malone KE, Saltzman BS, Daling JR. Risk of invasive breast carcinoma among women diagnosed with ductal carcinoma in situ and lobular carcinoma in situ, 1988–2001. Cancer. 2006; 106(10):2104–2112

[73] Brogi E, Murray MP, Corben AD. Lobular carcinoma, not only a classic. Breast J. 2010; 16 Suppl 1:S10–S14

[74] Rosen PP, Kosloff C, Lieberman PH, Adair F, Braun DW, Jr. Lobular carcinoma in situ of the breast. Detailed analysis of 99 patients with average follow-up of 24 years. Am J Surg Pathol. 1978; 2(3):225–251

[75] Port ER, Park A, Borgen PI, Morris E, Montgomery LL. Results of MRI screening for breast cancer in high-risk patients with LCIS and atypical hyperplasia. Ann Surg Oncol. 2007; 14 (3):1051–1057

[76] Sung JS, Malak SF, Bajaj P, Alis R, Dershaw DD, Morris EA. Screening breast MR imaging in women with a history of lobular carcinoma in situ. Radiology. 2011; 261(2):414–420

[77] Friedlander LC, Roth SO, Gavenonis SC. Results of MR imaging screening for breast cancer in high-risk patients with lobular carcinoma in situ. Radiology. 2011; 261(2):421–427

[78] Fisher B, Redmond C, Poisson R, et al. Eight-year results of a randomized clinical trial comparing total mastectomy and lumpectomy with or without irradiation in the treatment of breast cancer. N Engl J Med. 1989; 320 (13):822–828

[79] Dershaw DD, McCormick B, Osborne MP. Detection of local recurrence after conservative therapy for breast carcinoma. Cancer. 1992; 70(2):493–496

[80] Brennan S, Liberman L, Dershaw DD, Morris E. Breast MRI screening of women with a personal history of breast cancer. AJR Am J Roentgenol. 2010; 195(2):510–516

[81] Houssami N, Ciatto S, Martinelli F, Bonardi R, Duffy SW. Early detection of second breast cancers improves prognosis in breast cancer survivors. Ann Oncol. 2009; 20 (9):1505–1510

[82] Gweon HM, Cho N, Han W, et al. Breast MR imaging screening in women with a history of breast conservation therapy. Radiology. 2014; 272(2):366–373

[83] Yang TJ, Yang Q, Haffty BG, Moran MS. Prognosis for mammographically occult, early-stage breast cancer patients treated with breast-conservation therapy. Int J Radiat Oncol Biol Phys. 2010; 76(1):79–84

[84] Lehman CD, Lee JM, DeMartini WB, et al. Screening MRI in women with a personal history of breast cancer. J Natl Cancer Inst. 2016; 108(3):djv349

[85] Smith RA, Duffy SW, Tabár L. Breast cancer screening: the evolving evidence. Oncology (Williston Park). 2012; 26 (5):471–475, 479–481, 485–486

[86] Warner E, Hill K, Causer P, et al. Prospective study of breast cancer incidence in women with a BRCA1 or BRCA2 mutation under surveillance with and without magnetic resonance imaging. J Clin Oncol. 2011; 29(13):1664–1669

[87] Price ER, Hargreaves J, Lipson JA, et al. The California breast density information group: a collaborative response to the issues of breast density, breast cancer risk, and breast density notification legislation. Radiology. 2013; 269(3):887–892

[88] Berg WA, Blume JD, Cormack JB, et al. ACRIN 6666 Investigators. Combined screening with ultrasound and mammography vs mammography alone in women at elevated risk of breast cancer. JAMA. 2008; 299 (18):2151–2163

[89] Hooley RJ, Greenberg KL, Stackhouse RM, Geisel JL, Butler RS, Philpotts LE. Screening US in patients with mammographically dense breasts: initial experience with Connecticut Public Act 09–41. Radiology. 2012; 265(1):59–69

[90] Weigert J, Steenbergen S. The Connecticut experiments second year: ultrasound in the screening of women with dense breasts. Breast J. 2015; 21(2):175–180

[91] Sprague BL, Stout NK, Schechter C, et al. Benefits, harms, and cost-effectiveness of supplemental ultrasonography screening for women with dense breasts. Ann Intern Med. 2015; 162(3):157–166

[92] Kuhl CK, Schrading S, Strobel K, Schild HH, Hilgers RD, Bieling HB. Abbreviated breast magnetic resonance imaging (MRI): first postcontrast subtracted images and maximum-intensity projection-a novel approach to breast cancer screening with MRI. J Clin Oncol. 2014; 32(22):2304–2310

[93] Mango VL, Morris EA, David Dershaw D, et al. Abbreviated protocol for breast MRI: are multiple sequences needed for cancer detection? Eur J Radiol. 2015; 84 (1):65–70

3 Current Clinical Evidence on Abbreviated Breast Magnetic Resonance Imaging

Christiane Kuhl

3.1 The Need for Improved Breast Cancer Screening Methods

Irrespective of tumor biology, it is true that there is a close correlation between the stage of breast cancer at the time of diagnosis and cancer survival. Breast cancer is a highly curable disease if diagnosed at a stage where the disease is localized, that is, confined to the breast, with 10-year survival rates well above 95%. The prognosis is still good, with 10-year survival around 80%, if the disease is regional, that is, confined to the axillary lymph nodes. Yet once the disease has spread, that is, once distant metastases are present, survival rates will be greatly reduced, and the patient will usually die of the disease.[1]

The aim of screening is therefore to detect breast cancer in an early localized or regional stage. Mammographic screening has been found to be effective for this purpose, and helps reduce mortality from breast cancer.[2]

Some important reasons to search for breast cancer screening methods beyond mammography are overdiagnosis of biologically inert disease,[3] as well as underdiagnosis of prognostically important cancers that are observed with mammographic screening.

Overdiagnosis may be particularly problematic for structural (radiographic) breast imaging techniques, that is, mammography or tomosynthesis. Radiographic breast imaging detects cancer by depicting regressive changes such as tumor necrosis, apoptosis, or hypoxia—hallmarks of cancer that lead to the calcifications, fibrosis, and architectural distortions then picked up by a mammogram. It is well established that a screen-detected, that is, mammographically visible, breast cancer is associated with a better prognosis than a cancer of the same size that was not screen detected, that is, mammographically occult, but detected as so-called interval cancer in between mammographic screening rounds. This effect is referred to "length time bias." It implies that the cancer yield of mammographic screening may overestimate its power to reduce mortality because it detects prognostically less aggressive

types of breast cancer. Overdiagnosis—that is, the diagnosis of nonprogressive, self-limiting breast cancer—is a length time bias put to an extreme.

The flipside to this is that mammographic (or radiographic) imaging performs relatively poor in detecting rapidly growing, prognostically important breast cancers. Such cancers are usually not necessarily hypoxic, but well fed with nutrients and oxygen through active angiogenic activity; accordingly, they may not develop calcifications and do not induce fibrosis. Moreover, these cancers are usually hypercellular and exhibit pushing margins, which makes them mammographically occult if embedded in breast tissue, and even if they are mammographically detectable, they will be indistinguishable from cysts or fibroadenomas.

In summary, there is a propensity of radiographic imaging to detect slowly growing cancers, and a lack of sensitivity for prognostically important, rapidly growing, cancers.

The limited sensitivity of screening mammography has also been observed in DMIST (Digital Mammography Screening Trials). This trial was designed to compare the clinical performance of film-screen with that of digital mammography and recruited over 50,000 women. The DMIST found an overall sensitivity of screening mammography to range between 36% and 38% for women with dense breast tissue (ACR 3 and 4), suggesting that over half of cancers will not be picked up by screening mammography.[4]

Another piece of evidence on "underdiagnosis" is available through the performance reports on organized mammographic screening programs. European quality assurance guidelines accept an interval cancer rate (referenced to the background incidence of breast cancer) of up to 50% for 2-year screening periods. This implies that half of cancers that occur in a screening cohort will not be picked up by mammography.

Last, and most important, breast cancer continues to represent the most or second most important cause of cancer death, and is the main reason for "life years lost" in the female population. Despite several decades of publicly organized screening programs, breast cancer mortality remains high. This, together with the well-established correlation between early diagnosis and ultimate prognosis of women with breast cancer, suggests that there is room, and need, for further improvement of screening methods even for women at average risk.

3.2 Candidate Novel Breast Cancer Screening Methods

Current candidate methods for complementary breast cancer screening are digital breast tomosynthesis (DBT), contrast-enhanced spectral mammography (CESM), ultrasound, and magnetic resonance imaging (MRI).

Several large clinical studies have been published on the use of DBT for supplementary breast cancer screening, that is, the use of DBT in addition to screening mammography. The added cancer yield achievable by DBT ranges between 1.1 and 6.7 per 1,000 women, with an average of 1.25 per 1,000. The main impact of using DBT in addition to mammography is to avoid recall and improve the Positive Predictive Value (PPV) of biopsy recommendations from 23% to 29%. Accordingly, DBT will modestly improve cancer detection rates / sensitivity, as well as specificity / PPVs.[11,12,13] However, information on the biologic profile of the breast cancers that were found by DBT in addition to mammographic screening is scarce. Technically, DBT mainly improves the detection of architectural distortions and stellate lesions—cancers that, based on their imaging phenotype, may more likely represent well-differentiated, low-grade, disease. As such, although DBT may avoid some "underdiagnosis" of breast cancer, that is, will improve the detection of breast cancer missed by regular full-field digital mammography, it is relatively unlikely that it will help reduce overdiagnosis. Indeed, for

reasons mentioned earlier, it is possible that it will even contribute to additional overdiagnosis of biologically unimportant disease (▶ Table 3.1).

CESM has so far been used for diagnostic purposes only, not for screening. However, the emerging results suggest that contrast injection may greatly increase the sensitivity of digital mammography, to levels that may be similar to those obtained with contrast-enhanced breast MRI. Although sensitivity levels are still a matter under investigation, it is likely that CESM could serve as surrogate for diagnostic breast MRI. If one considers using CESM for screening, it is important to keep in mind that the safety profile of any type of iodinated contrast agent used for CESM is far less advantageous compared to that observed for any type of MRI contrast agent used for breast MRI. With modern, macrocyclic contrast agents recommended for breast MRI, the volume of injection ranges between 5 and 9 mL, whereas the injection volume for iodinated contrast agents for CESM ranges between 70 and 150 mL. Although nephrogenic systemic fibrosis (NFS) screening may be recommendable in some women prior to injection of a macrocyclic MRI contrast agent, it will always be important to test for renal as well as thyroid function in women undergoing injection of iodinated contrast agents. Accordingly, patient preparation will be more complex for CESM, especially if this method was used in a screening situation.

Ultrasound has been proposed to help improve the detection of breast cancer in women with dense radiographic tissue (▶ Table 3.2). Several prospective screening studies showed that screening ultrasound is indeed useful to increase the cancer detection rate by an average of 4.1 per

Table 3.1 Evidence on the use of digital breast tomosynthesis for screening purposes

Author	Year	Journal	No. of participants	Additional cancer yield
Rose et al[5]	2013	AJR	9.499	1.1/1,000 (not significant)
Ciatto et al[6]	2013	Lancet Oncology	7.292	2.7/1,000
Skaane et al[7]	2013	Radiology	12.621	2.3/1,000
Friedewald et al[8]	2014	JAMA	454.850	1.2/1,000
Sharpe et al[9]	2015	Radiology	5.703	1.9/1,000
McDonald et al[10]	2015	AJR	15.571	1.3/1,000
Average additional cancer yield				1.25/1,000

Table 3.2 Evidence on the use of breast ultrasound for screening

Type	Author	Year	Women	Added cancers	Additional cancer yield	Fraction of DCIS	PPV
HH-US	Gordon et al[12]	1995	12.706	44	3.5 per 1,000	0 (0%)	16.0%
HH-US	Buchberger et al[13]	2000	8.103	32	3.9 per 1,000	5 (13%)	9.0%
HH-US	Kaplan et al[14]	2001	1.862	6	3.0 per 1,000	1 (16%)	10.0%
HH-US	Kolb et al[15]	2002	13.547	37	2.7 per 1,000	1 (3%)	10.0%
HH-US	Crystal et al[16]	2003	1.517	7	4.6 per 1,000	0 (0%)	18.0%
HH-US	Berg et al[17]	2008	2.809	41	4.5 per 1000	1 (2%)	8.0%
HH-US	Ohuchi et al[18]	2015	36.859	61	1.7 per 1,000	9 (15%)	9.7%
ABVS	Brem et al[19]	2015	15.318	30	1.9 per 1,000	2 (7%)	9.8%

Abbreviations: ABVS, automated breast volume scanner; DCIS, ductal carcinoma in situ; HH-US, handheld breast ultrasound; PPV, positive predictive value.

1,000 compared with mammographic screening in the same individuals. The increased cancer detection rate associated with supplemental ultrasound screening does reduce the interval cancer rate. In their American College of Radiology Imaging Network (ACRIN)–sponsored 6666 trial,[21] Berg and colleagues reported an interval cancer rate as low as 8%. A limitation of screening ultrasound is the relatively broad overlap of ultrasound imaging features of benign and malignant lesions. Published rates of PPV for screening ultrasound range between 8 and just over 20%.[22] This may lead to substantial additional downstream costs and possibly morbidity. Another limitation is the radiologist's time it takes to complete a screening ultrasound study. In the 6666 trial by Berg and colleagues,[21] the average time for a bilateral ultrasound screening study was around 19 minutes. Automated breast ultrasound may help reduce the physician time substantially; however, at the time this article was written, the supplemental cancer yield and PPV rates of screening by automated breast ultrasound was unknown.[23]

After completion of their ACRIN 6666 ultrasound screening study, Berg and coworkers were able to offer their screening cohort—women who had undergone several years of annual mammography plus ultrasound—a single round of screening MRI. This yielded an additional supplemental cancer detection rate of 14.6 per 1,000, which compares favorably to the rate of 4.1 per 1,000 in the same cohort based on mammography plus ultrasound screening.[24] This evidence is in good agreement with a series of studies that had been published on the use of MRI, mammography, and ultrasound for screening women at increased risk of breast cancer, and which consistently found about doubled sensitivity of MRI compared with the combined use of mammography and ultrasound.[25,26,27,28,29,30,31,32,33,34,35,36]

Beyond the comparison of mere numbers of "cancers detected" by different breast screening methods, it is more and more evident that it is at least as important to investigate what type of cancers are diagnosed by different screening methods. The major difference between conventional breast imaging or ultrasound and breast MRI is the fact that in the latter case, cancer is detected due to its local contrast enhancement. Breast MRI is not only a diagnostic tool but also an in vivo imaging biomarker for disease activity or tumor biology. Enhancement of a ductal carcinoma in situ (DCIS) or of an invasive cancer requires a locally increased vessel density, an increased vessel permeability and—in the case of DCIS—an increased permeability of the ductal basal membrane. Breast cancer detection in MRI is therefore based on pathophysiological changes that are indicative of cancer proliferation, infiltrative growth, and metastasis.[37,38]

In good agreement with these pathophysiological considerations, it has been shown that screening MRI is associated with something one could call a "reverse length time bias," that is, cancer detection in MRI is biased toward prognostically important disease. Cancers detected only by MRI tend to exhibit high nuclear grade and high Ki-67 values, hallmarks of rapid growth. In turn, malignant lesions that went undetected by MRI screening, and picked up by mammography alone, typically consist of low-grade DCIS. Trials that compared the added value of mammography in women undergoing MRI for screening concordantly found that the additional cancers diagnosed through mammographic screening mainly represent disease with limited, if any, prognostic importance.

3.3 Evidence for the Use of Breast MRI for Screening

The American Cancer Society guidelines recommend annual breast MRI for screening of women at an increased risk of breast cancer, defined as a 20% lifetime risk.[39] Many women will carry such a lifetime risk, yet only a minority of women who would need MRI for screening do indeed have access to MRI screening.[40] This is not because the respective MR systems would not be physically available.[41] Although the individual reasons for failure to undergo MRI screening for women at high risk of breast cancer are not well established, the perceived high cost of the examination, together with a lack of knowledge about the implications of a high lifetime risk, will play a major role.

Trials that compared the diagnostic accuracy of MRI with that of screening mammography with or without ultrasound (▶ Table 3.3) yielded concordant results in that MRI was consistently more accurate than mammography and ultrasound. The actual sensitivity levels achieved by MRI varied between 71% and 100% in the different studies. The major reason for sensitivity levels below 80% observed in some of the early studies on MRI screening was failure to diagnose DCIS on MRI. Later publications by the same groups confirmed this. Accordingly, the sensitivity of MRI will range between 90 and 100%. Cancers missed by MRI are, in the vast majority of cases, due to low-risk (low-grade) DCIS.[42]

The EVAluation of imaging methods for early diagnosis of familial breast cancer, or EVA trial, investigated the respective contributions of mammography, ultrasound, and MRI to the individual diagnosis of breast cancer in intermediate- to high-risk women undergoing screening and found that MRI is by far the most important single imaging method. In the EVA cohort, mammography alone exhibited an average sensitivity of just above 33%, which is in good concordance with the mammographic sensitivity established in the DMIST trial for women with intermediately dense and dense breast tissue. If ultrasound was added to mammography, the sensitivity rose by about 50% to an overall sensitivity of 48%. MRI alone offered a sensitivity of 93%. If mammography was added to MRI, there was a nonsignificant increase in sensitivity to 100%. The additional lesions depicted by mammography, that is, lesions that had been undetected by MRI, were three cases of low-grade DCIS. Accordingly, the results of the EVA trial suggested that (1) MRI could be used as a stand-alone imaging method and (2) the cancers missed by MRI represent cancers which could well be considered "insignificant." The EVA trial thus provided initial evidence for the fact that MRI could avoid not only underdiagnosis of biologically important invasive disease, but also overdiagnosis due to diagnosis of low-grade DCIS.

The appropriate metric to rate the success of breast cancer screening programs is the interval cancer rate observed in the screened cohort. In the different MRI screening cohorts, the reported interval cancer rates ranged between 0% and 6%. Accordingly, this rate is much lower than that observed in regular mammographic screening programs, where interval cancer rates as high as 50% have been reported. The low interval cancer rate observed in MRI screening trials was specifically remarkable in view of the high risk of the women included in the MRI screening trials; women with familial breast cancer tend to develop rapidly growing cancers. The higher the rate of cancers with fast growth, the more difficult it is to achieve low interval cancer rates.

It should be well understood that, due to the frequently "atypical" imaging appearance of *BRCA*-associated breast cancers, and the high prevalence of benign enhancing lesions observed in young women at high risk, MRI screening of these women belongs to the most demanding applications of breast MRI in general. Profound personal experience with breast MRI in general, and with diagnosis of familial breast cancer in particular, is of utmost

Table 3.3 Evidence on the use of magnetic resonance imaging (MRI) for screening

	Riedl et al[32]	Sardanelli et al[31]	Kuhl et al[30]	Lehmann et al[36]	Sardanelli et al[31]	Hagen et al	Kuhl et al[29]	Leach et al[27]	Kriegeet al	Warner et al[28]	Morris et al[25]	Stoutjesdijk et al	Kuhl et al
Study period	1999–2011	2000–2007	2002–2005	2005	2000–2003	2002–2006	1996–2002	1997–2004	1999–2002	1997–2003	2000–2001	1994–2001	1996–1998
No. of participants	559	501	687	195	278	491	529	648	1.909	256	367	139	192
Women years	1.365	1.592	1.679	195	377	867	1.542	1.881	5.249	457	n.a.	258	419
No. of cancers	40	52	27	6	18	21	43	35	44	22	14	10	9
"Minimal cancers"	68%	56%	81%	83%	44%	43%	58%	46%	43%	9%	64%	50%	22%
Rate of positive lymph node	8%	25%	11%	17%	17%	29%	16%	19%	14%	9%	4%	30%	0%
Sensitivity MRI	90%	91%	93%	100%	94%	86%	93%	77%	71%	77%	100%	100%	100%
Sensitivity mammography	37.5%	50%	33%	33%	59%	48%	33%	40%	40%	36%	0%	46%	33%
Sensitivity ultrasound	37.5%	52	37%	17%	65%	n.a.	40%	n.a.	n.a.	33%	n.a.	n.a.	33%
PPV MRI	20%	65%	48%	43%	63%	n.a.	50%	7%	30%	49%	17%	38%	64%
PPV Mx	28%	71%	39%	50%	77%	n.a.	23%	10%	58%	83%	n.a.	33%	30%
PPV US	27%	62%	33%	25%	65%	n.a.	11%	n.a.	n.a.	23%	n.a.	n.a.	14%

Abbreviations: n.a., not available; PPV, positive predictive value; US, ultrasound.

importance. It is important to realize that, as with all imaging methods, a learning curve exists for breast MRI as well that needs to be taken into consideration when reviewing published results on MRI screening. This is also true for the PPV; recent trials suggest that the PPV of MRI, if used for screening, is at least as high as that of mammographic screening in the same individuals.[43,44]

3.4 The Rationale and Concept of "Abbreviated Breast MRI"

The rationale of "abbreviated breast MRI" (AB-MRI) is to reduce the image acquisition time, thus the magnet time, of breast MRI, as well as the image reviewing time, thus the radiologist time, needed for breast MRI interpretation (▶ Fig. 3.1). The aim is to reduce the cost associated with a breast MRI screening study, as well as to improve patients' (or, rather, women's) acceptance of breast MRI. The overall goal is to improve access to breast MRI for screening not only for women at high and intermediate risk, but also for those at average risk who wish to undergo screening with a test that grants the highest cancer detection rate that is currently achievable.

The concept of AB-MRI was introduced by our group[45] and consists of the following four components:

1. Acquire an abbreviated breast MRI protocol that lasts no longer than 5 minutes magnet time.
2. Use maximum intensity projection (MIP) reconstructions of the first postcontrast subtracted

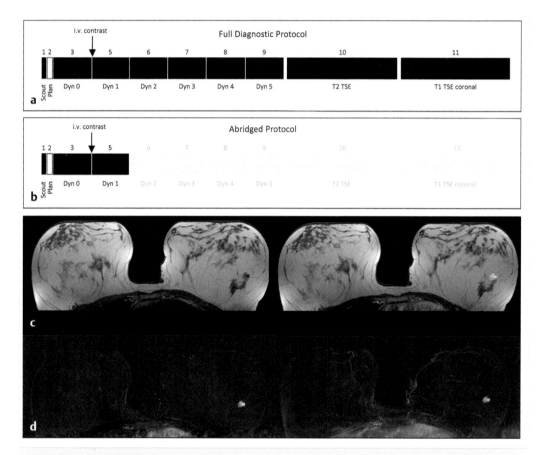

Fig. 3.1 Concept of abbreviated breast magnetic resonance imaging (MRI). **(a)** Schematic presentation of the abbreviated and the full diagnostic protocol. B-E MR images of a patient with left-sided breast cancer. **(b)** Midbreast section of the baseline (precontrast) dynamic acquisition (Dyn 0 in **a**). **(c)** Corresponding section of the first postcontrast dynamic acquisition (Dyn 1 in **a**). **(d)** Corresponding FAST (first postcontrast subtracted) image, generated by subtracting image **(b)** from image **(c)**. E, maximum intensity projection (MIP), generated by fusing all FAST sections into a single 3D-like projection image.

(FAST) images for quick review and to decide upon the presence or absence of significant enhancement.

3. Use the individual FAST images and, if necessary, their nonsubtracted pre- and postcontrast source images, for characterization of enhancing lesions.
4. Have expert radiologists with specific expertise in breast MRI as well as in reading AB-MRI interpret the images.

Complying with each of these components is essential to reproduce the results published by our group. Personal experiences with reading abbreviated protocols are easy to establish. A possibility is to prospectively read a larger number of MRI screening studies and review the first postcontrast series only. Details on acquisition protocols and interpretation guidelines will be discussed in Chapter 4 of this book.

The usual, multiparametric, "full protocol" breast MRI provides information on high-resolution, cross-sectional lesion morphology, as well as functional information on a variety of tissue features. This includes information on tissue microvessel and macrovessel perfusion, vessel permeability, tissue relaxation times, tissue cellularity/proliferation rate, and interstitial pressure. All this information can be useful for tissue characterization, that is, for the distinction of benign versus malignant lesions, as well as for a further classification of the biologic and prognostic importance of breast cancers and their precursors (DCIS). Due to its complexity, its diagnostic power, and its cost, MRI has traditionally been used as a third-line imaging method, that is, done in patients in whom disease was already known to be present on clinical grounds or based on other imaging methods, and where an improved differential diagnosis or diagnosis of disease stage was desired.

Accordingly, when breast MRI was developed in the 1990s, it had mainly been used to settle equivocal conventional imaging results and/or on patients with known breast cancer in whom an accurate delineation of extent or an accurate classification of disease was desired, or for response assessment. In such situations, it is appropriate to employ extensive pulse sequence protocols in order to achieve a maximum diagnostic accuracy for disease characterization (differentiation of benign vs. malignant disease and also assessment of cancer viability). Accordingly, current breast MRI protocols are time consuming to acquire and to read. A typical MRI study occupies the MR system for up to 40 minutes and generates several hundred images.

Mammographic screening, on the other hand, is a highly standardized and relatively simple procedure. Women undergo mammography, usually without clinical examination, and the resulting mammograms are interpreted by highly trained and specialized screening radiologists who batch read up to 100 mammograms per hour.

Accordingly, we proposed to use an approach to breast MRI screening that pursues a concept similar to that of mammographic screening programs. We proposed an abbreviated, short MRI protocol that is limited to the early postcontrast period, then to use standard image reconstruction tools (subtraction and MIP) to allow a very fast reading of these abbreviated protocols, and to compensate for the reduction of imaging information by having expert radiologists interpret this limited protocol. The aim was to substantially reduce image acquisition and reading time of screening MRI. Long-term goal is to increase the access to screening breast MRI.

The rationale to focus on the early postcontrast period is as follows. The principal concept of dynamic contrast-enhanced breast MRI is to detect cancer based on their enhancement that will be faster and stronger compared with that of the adjacent fibroglandular tissue. Invasive breast cancers usually reach their maximal enhancement already in the early postcontrast period; this is then followed by either a plateau of enhancement or even a signal loss (washout). As opposed to this, benign changes as well as the background enhancement of the normal fibroglandular tissue will exhibit persistent enhancement, that is, it will become progressively brighter over time. Accordingly, the optimal contrast between a cancer and its environment is achieved in the very early postcontrast phase, where contrast enhancement in the cancer is maximal, and where signal of benign changes is still minimal.

Accordingly, the early postcontrast phase is best suitable to detect significant enhancement, and also to characterize enhancing lesions based on their morphology. Anatomic details such as fine spiculations are best resolved when the contrast between the cancer and its surrounding tissue is optimal. The abbreviated protocol published by us consists of only one post-contrast phase; however, it does provide information on enhancement kinetics. Because images are acquired in the early post-contrast phase, AB-MRI captures the wash-in kinetics. With abbreviated protocols, we may lose the information on wash-out kinetics that is assessed through review of the additional dynamic frames. Yet while wash-out kinetics were essential in the early days of breast MRI, their importance was decreasing with the increasing spatial resolution that can be established with contemporary MR pulse sequences, and which improves the analysis of morphological details of enhancing lesions.

Our regular breast MRI protocol, as well as the abbreviated protocol, consists of a dynamic series acquired without fat suppression, as detailed in Chapter 4. ▶ Fig. 3.2 demonstrates how we use non–fat-suppressed images to improve the depiction of anatomic details of enhancing lesions detected on FAST images.

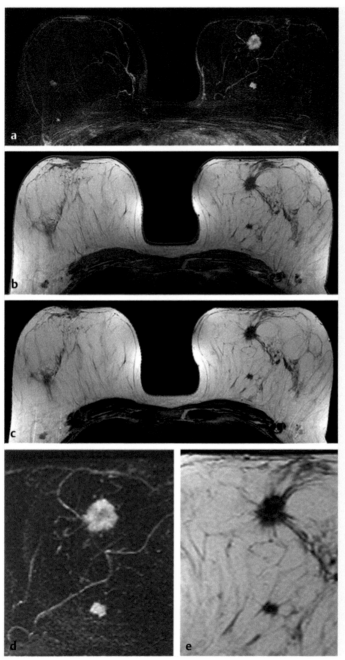

Fig. 3.2 A 62-year-old patient with mammographically visible suspicious mass in her left breast. (**a**) Maximum intensity projection (MIP) image displaying two enhancing masses in the left breast, (**b**) corresponding precontrast non–fat-suppressed nonsubtracted image, (**c**) corresponding non–fat-suppressed T2-weighted turbo spin-echo (TSE) image, (**d**) close-up view of the FAST image (**a**), (**e**) close-up view of the precontrast non–fat-suppressed image (**b**). Note the crisp contrast between the enhancing lesion and the breast parenchyma. Note that the small cancer toward the chest wall appears well circumscribed, lobulated on the subtracted image. Note that the unenhanced, non–fat-suppressed images display the irregular borders and spiculations better than the enhanced, subtracted images. This is multifocal invasive breast cancer on the left. Enhancing lesion in the right breast, lateral quadrant, was not called.

3.5 Diagnostic Accuracy of AB-MRI Screening Compared with Full-Protocol Breast MRI

To investigate the diagnostic accuracy that is achievable with such an abbreviated protocol, and to compare its utility with that obtained with a full, routine breast MRI protocol in the same women, we conducted a prospective reader study. We recruited 443 women who underwent a total 606 MRI screening rounds over 18 months with the AB-MRI and the full breast MRI screening protocol. The abbreviated protocol consisted of only one pre- and one postcontrast acquisition, plus the respective FAST images and their MIP reconstruction. Women at moderately to mildly increased risk were offered MRI for screening only if they had undergone two view digital mammography, double read by two experienced breast radiologists with negative or benign results, as well as a high-resolution ultrasound screening study of the breast, conducted by dedicated breast radiologist, again with negative or benign results.

In the 606 screening rounds, a total of 11 breast cancers were found by MRI; in another 8 women, high-risk lesions (i.e., atypical ductal hyperplasia [ADH], lobular intraepithelial neoplasia [LIN]) were identified on MRI. Of the breast cancers, four (36%) were in the intraductal stage and seven (64%) were invasive, with a median size of 8 mm. As was expected on pathophysiological grounds, distribution of nuclear grading of cancers and DCIS was skewed to a higher than normal prevalence of high-grade disease (57%). Since all participants had had a normal mammogram at the time of study inclusion, this translates into an additional (supplementary) cancer yield of 18.3 per 1,000 women.

We had anticipated that an abbreviated protocol, that is, withholding diagnostic information, should be associated with a reduced diagnostic accuracy, but suspected that it may be acceptable to give up some of the very high sensitivity and specificity of regular screening breast MRI, and trade it for acquisition and interpretation speed. However, we found that the diagnostic accuracy of the AB-MRI screening protocol was indeed comparable or even identical to that of our routine breast MRI screening protocol. Even with a quick review of the MIP images, presence of breast cancer could be excluded with a negative predicative value (NPV) of 99.8%. One of the 11 breast cancers (a small, 4-mm lobular-invasive cancer) was not prospectively identified on the MIP image, but only on the FAST image. This suggests that, until more experiences with AB-MRI exist, review of FAST images is recommendable even if the MIP image does not reveal significant enhancement. If FAST images were used for analysis, all cancers were correctly identified. FAST images were also useful to correctly characterize enhancing areas that were identified on MIP images. Accordingly, with the abbreviated protocol, the same added cancer yield was achieved as with the regular screening breast MRI protocol, that is, sensitivity was equal to that of the full diagnostic protocol.

A total of 53 women received a "BIRADS3 diagnosis" based on the reading of the abbreviated protocol. In almost half of them, that is, 20/53, the lesion that had been categorized as "probably benign" was downgraded to a BIRADS2 category when the full diagnostic protocol was reviewed. Since a BIRADS3 diagnosis is usually managed by short-term follow-up, whereas a BIRADS2 diagnosis does not require additional imaging, this is of relevance with regard to patient management. On the other hand, in four of the same 53 women, reading the full diagnostic protocol caused an "upgrading" of the respective lesions to BIRADS4, such that these women underwent MR-guided biopsy for clarification; none of these women were finally found to have breast cancer.

Accordingly, overall, the usefulness of additional pulse sequences for definitive noninvasive characterization of enhancing lesions detected on the abbreviated protocol is limited. Therefore, in our practice, if we use an abbreviated protocol clinically and detect an equivocal enhancing lesions, we would not re-invite the patient to come back and undergo the full protocol. Rather, we proceed as with lesions detected on full-protocol MRI, that is, do a second-look ultrasound at the site of the MRI abnormality, and, if no clearly benign correlate is identified, we proceed to MR-guided biopsy right away.

The PPV3 (positive predictive value of biopsies performed) of 24.4% for AB-MRI in an average-risk screening setting is comparable to the PPV3 observed after digital mammography or DBT. Of note, however, there is no such thing as "recall" and "diagnostic assessment" after a screening AB-MRI study—all MRI diagnoses are final. Costs associated with recall after screening mammography are important drivers of the overall costs of a mammographic screening program. Since AB-MRI works without recall, this needs to be considered for a full-cost accounting of mammographic versus AB-MRI screening.

3.6 Time to Perform and Read Abbreviated Breast MRI

The abbreviated protocol allowed a substantial reduction of image acquisition time. Whereas the regular breast MRI protocol consisted of 10 pulse sequences covering an acquisition time of almost 20 minutes, the abbreviated protocol took about 3 minutes table time. This included a fast localizer, a reference scan needed for preparing subsequent parallel imaging, and one pre- and one postcontrast acquisition. Moreover, and at least as important, the reading time was very short for the images of the abbreviated protocol. Expert radiologists took less than 3 seconds for establishing presence or absence of significant enhancement based on the single MIP image. In case radiologists did identify significant enhancement, they took under 30 seconds to interpret the individual FAST images.

Since, in a screening cohort, the vast majority of women will not exhibit significant enhancement, the velocity with which a radiologist is able to determine absence of breast cancer will be the most important driver of overall radiologist time (and, thus, cost). Since, with AB-MRI, such absence of breast cancer will be established on the basis of the MIP readings, these very fast readings will be sufficient for the majority of cases.

AB-MRI reading times compare favorably with the time needed even for batch reading of organized mammographic mass screening programs, where a reading or interpretation times of about 60 seconds are allotted per screening case (four mammograms). The reason for the extreme speed with which AB-MRI studies can be read is the fact that FAST images as well as their MIPs provide high-contrast images. There is no actual "search" for a breast cancer. Enhancing areas are easily detectable; the actual task of a radiologist is not to detect, but to characterize enhancement. This is quite unlike the situation in mammographic screening where, for the majority of women with noninvoluted breasts, mammograms provide low-contrast images, where the main task of a radiologist is, first, to search for subtle changes that may be a correlate of breast cancer growth.

With the very short magnet time of abbreviated MRI, it may become conceivable to complete AB-MRI screening studies within a 5-minute magnet time. This, in turn, means that dedicated MR systems are now needed that are optimized for high-volume screening applications. Specifically, this implies that scanners should be built that are optimized for prone imaging, and that allow fast patient throughput. All in all, the use of MRI for breast cancer screening on even a population-wide scale seems attainable if abbreviated protocols and dedicated breast MR systems become available.

3.6.1 Emerging Results of Other Groups

In the last 2 years, a couple of further studies have been published that adopted the concept of AB-MRI. Unfortunately, however, the definition of what constitutes "abbreviated" varies between authors. Variable protocols have been published, with the common denominator being the fact that authors reduced their regular pulse sequence protocol to a variable extent. The suggestion to use MIP images for detection of significant contrast enhancement, then individual first postcontrast subtracted images for characterization—an important pillar of the concept of AB-MRI as proposed by us—has not been pursued by other groups thus far. Chapter 4 will provide detailed information on how to conduct and interpret an abbreviated breast MRI study with the technique proposed by us.

Mango et al[46] in 2015 conducted a study on the utility of abbreviated protocol for breast cancer detection in 100 consecutive breast MR imaging studies with biopsy-proven unilateral breast cancer (79% invasive, 21% DCIS). Four readers evaluated only the first postcontrast T1-weighted image and its subtraction as well as the respective MIP. Results were compared with their standard pulse sequence protocol consisting of 13 pulse sequences plus post-processed images. Average sensitivity across the four readers was 96%. In good agreement with the experiences published in our paper,[32] the authors concluded that one pre- and one postcontrast acquisition may be sufficient for establishing the diagnosis of breast cancer. The average time to read was 44 seconds for the abbreviated protocol.

Grimm et al[47] in 2015 conducted a multireader study on two different abbreviated protocols on a total of 48 patients with 12 breast cancers. Protocol 1 consisted of fatsat T2-weighted imaging, followed by one pre- and the first postcontrast T1-weighted acquisition. Protocol 2 consisted of protocol 1 images plus a second postcontrast acquisition. The respective full protocols consisted of additional non–fatsat T1-weighted imaging, fatsat T2-weighted imaging, and additional post-contrast dynamic acquisitions. Although the authors did not report on a statistically significant difference of cancer detection rate (sensitivity), they do report a similar, yet overall relatively low diagnostic accuracy for abbreviated as well as for the full diagnostic protocol.

Moschetta et al[48] in 2016 conducted a study on 470 patients undergoing breast MRI for a variety of clinical indications (screening, staging, problem-solving). In the cohort, they observed a total 185 breast lesions in 177 patients. The term "abbreviated" in this study was used to denote that the respective pulse sequence was somewhat shorter than the one used on a regular basis by the same group. The protocol consisted of a STIR, a T2w-TSE, and one pre- and one postcontrast T1-weighted acquisition. The authors found a sensitivity, specificity, PPV, and NPV that was equivalent for the "abbreviated" and regular full protocol.

Harvey et al[50] conducted a study on the use of abbreviated protocols for high-risk screening. Their regular breast MRI protocol took 30 minutes to acquire, while the "abbreviated" version took just over 10 minutes. They reported on an interpretation time of 1.55 minutes for the abbreviated protocol, compared with 6.43 minutes for the full protocol. They found equivalent diagnostic accuracy of the abbreviated versus the full protocol and explained that changes of patient management were observed in 12 out of 568 MRI studies (2.1%).

In their study on the utility of AB-MRI protocol for local staging of known breast cancers, Heacock et al[49] read MRI studies of 107 biopsy-proven breast cancers with an abbreviated protocol consisting of T1-weighted pre- and postcontrast and subtracted images (protocol 1 without clinical information, protocol 2 with clinical information), and after adding T2-weighted images (protocol 3) by three readers. They found a detection rate of 97.8, 99.4, and 99.4% for the three protocols. They concluded that T2-weighted imaging did not improve detection rate—thus confirming the approach pursued by our group—and confirmed that AB-MRI has a high rate of cancer detection.

All in all, in spite of the variability of pulse sequence design, the results published by different groups are quite consistent in that the abbreviated protocol was shown to offer equivalent cancer detection rates and diagnostic accuracy compared with the authors' respective full protocols.

References

[1] Cancer Stat Facts: Female Breast Cancer. seer.cancer.gov/statfacts/html/breast.html
[2] Kaplan HG, Malmgren JA, Atwood MK, Calip GS. Cancer. 2015; 121:2553–2556
[3] Morris E, Feig SA, Drexler M, Lehman C. Implications of Overdiagnosis: Impact on Screening Mammography Practices. Popul Health Manag. 2015; 18 Suppl 1:S3–S11
[4] Pisano ED, Gatsonis C, Hendrick E, et al. Digital Mammographic Imaging Screening Trial (DMIST) Investigators Group. Diagnostic performance of digital versus film mammography for breast-cancer screening. N Engl J Med. 2005; 353 (17):1773–1783
[5] Rose SL, Tidwell AL, Bujnoch LJ, Kushwaha AC, Nordmann AS, Sexton R, Jr. Implementation of breast tomosynthesis in a routine screening practice: an observational study. AJR Am J Roentgenol. 2013; 200:1401–1408
[6] Ciatto S, Houssami N, Bernardi D, et al. Integration of 3D digital mammography with tomosynthesis for population breast-cancer screening (STORM): a prospective comparison study. Lancet Oncol. 2013; 14:583–589
[7] Skaane P, Bandos AI, Eben EB, et al. Two-view digital breast tomosynthesis screening with synthetically reconstructed projection images: comparison with digital breast tomosynthesis with full-field digital mammographic images. Radiology. 2014; 271(3):655–663
[8] Friedewald SM, Rafferty EA, Rose SL, et al. Breast cancer screening using tomosynthesis in combination with digital mammography. JAMA. 2014; 311(24):2499–2507
[9] Sharpe RE, Jr, Venkataraman S, Phillips J, et al. Increased Cancer Detection Rate and Variations in the Recall Rate Resulting from Implementation of 3D Digital Breast Tomosynthesis into a Population-based Screening Program. Radiology. 2016; 278:698–706
[10] McDonald ES, McCarthy AM, Akhtar AL, Synnestvedt MB, Schnall M, Conant EF. Baseline Screening Mammography: Performance of Full-Field Digital Mammography Versus Digital Breast Tomosynthesis. AJR Am J Roentgenol. 2015; 205:1143–1148
[11] Gilbert FJ, Tucker L, Young KC. Digital breast tomosynthesis (DBT): a review of the evidence for use as a screening tool. Clin Radiol. 2016; 71(2):141–150
[12] Gordon PB, Goldenberg SL. Malignant breast masses detected only by ultrasound. A retrospective review. Cancer. 1995; 76:626–630
[13] Buchberger W, Niehoff A, Obrist P, DeKoekkoek, -Doll P, Dünser M. Clinically and mammographically occult breast lesions: detection and classification with high-resolution sonography. Semin Ultrasound CT MR. 2000; 21:325–336
[14] Kaplan SS. Clinical utility of bilateral whole-breast US in the evaluation of women with dense breast tissue. Radiology. 2001; 221:641–649
[15] Kolb TM, Lichy J, Newhouse JH. Comparison of the performance of screening mammography, physical examination, and breast US and evaluation of factors that influence them: an analysis of 27,825 patient evaluations. Radiology. 2002; 225:165–175
[16] Crystal P, Strano SD, Shcharynski S, Koretz MJ. Using sonography to screen women with mammographically dense breasts. AJR Am J Roentgenol. 2003; 181:177–182
[17] Berg WA, Blume JD, Cormack JB, et al. ACRIN 6666 Investigators. Combined screening with ultrasound and mammography vs mammography alone in women at elevated risk of breast cancer. JAMA. 2008; 299:2151–2163

[18] Ohuchi N, Suzuki A, Sobue T, et al. J-START investigator groups. Sensitivity and specificity of mammography and adjunctive ultrasonography to screen for breast cancer in the Japan Strategic Anti-cancer Randomized Trial (J-START): a randomised controlled trial. Lancet. 2016; 387:341–348

[19] Brem RF, Tabár L, Duffy SW, et al. Assessing improvement in detection of breast cancer with three-dimensional automated breast US in women with dense breast tissue: the SomoInsight Study. Radiology. 2015; 274:663–673

[20] Schrading S, Kuhl CK. Mammographic, US, and MR imaging phenotypes of familial breast cancer. Radiology. 2008; 246:58–70

[21] Berg WA, Blume JD, Cormack JB, et al. ACRIN 6666 Investigators. Combined screening with ultrasound and mammography vs mammography alone in women at elevated risk of breast cancer. JAMA. 2008; 299(18):2151–2163

[22] Melnikow J, Fenton JJ, Whitlock EP, et al. Supplemental Screening for Breast Cancer in Women With Dense Breasts: A Systematic Review for the U.S. Preventive Services Task Force. Ann Intern Med. 2016; •; ••. DOI: 10.7326/M15–1789

[23] Kelly KM, Dean J, Lee SJ, Comulada WS. Breast cancer detection: radiologists' performance using mammography with and without automated whole-breast ultrasound. Eur Radiol. 2010; 20(11):2557–2564

[24] Berg WA, Zhang Z, Lehrer D, et al. ACRIN 6666 Investigators. Detection of breast cancer with addition of annual screening ultrasound or a single screening MRI to mammography in women with elevated breast cancer risk. JAMA. 2012; 307 (13):1394–1404

[25] Morris EA, Liberman L, Ballon DJ, et al. MRI of occult breast carcinoma in a high-risk population. AJR Am J Roentgenol. 2003; 181(3):619–626

[26] Kriege M, Brekelmans CT, Boetes C, et al. Magnetic Resonance Imaging Screening Study Group. Efficacy of MRI and mammography for breast-cancer screening in women with a familial or genetic predisposition. N Engl J Med. 2004; 351 (5):427–437

[27] Leach MO, Boggis CR, Dixon AK, et al. Screening with magnetic resonance imaging and mammography of a UK population at high familial risk of breast cancer: a prospective multicentre cohort study (MARIBS). Lancet. 2005; 365 (9473):1769–1778

[28] Warner E, Plewes DB, Hill KA, et al. Surveillance of BRCA1 and BRCA2 mutation carriers with magnetic resonance imaging, ultrasound, mammography, and clinical breast examination. JAMA. 2004; 292(11):1317–1325

[29] Kuhl CK, Schrading S, Leutner CC, et al. Mammography, breast ultrasound, and magnetic resonance imaging for surveillance of women at high familial risk for breast cancer. J Clin Oncol. 2005; 23(33):8469–8476

[30] Kuhl C, Weigel S, Schrading S, et al. Prospective multicenter cohort study to refine management recommendations for women at elevated familial risk of breast cancer: the EVA trial. J Clin Oncol. 2010; 28(9):1450–1457

[31] Sardanelli F, Podo F, Santoro F, et al. Multicenter surveillance of women at high genetic breast cancer risk using mammography, ultrasonography, and contrast-enhanced magnetic resonance imaging (the high breast cancer risk italian 1 study): final results. Invest Radiol. 2011; 46(2):94–105

[32] Riedl CC, Luft N, Bernhart C, et al. 2014

[33] Sung JS, Lee CH, Morris EA, Oeffinger KC, Dershaw DD. Screening breast MR imaging in women with a history of chest irradiation. Radiology. 2011; 259(1):65–71

[34] Sung JS, Malak SF, Bajaj P, Alis R, Dershaw DD, Morris EA. 2011. DOI: 10.1148/radiol.11110091

[35] Port ER, Park A, Borgen PI, Morris E, Montgomery LL. Results of MRI screening for breast cancer in high-risk patients with LCIS and atypical hyperplasia. Ann Surg Oncol. 2007; 14 (3):1051–1057

[36] Lehman CD, Lee JM, DeMartini WB, Hippe DS, Rendi MH, Kalish G, Porter P, Gralow J, Partridge SC. 2016. DOI: 10.1093/. DOI: jnci. DOI: /djv349

[37] Kuhl CK. Why do purely intraductal cancers enhance on breast MR images? Radiology. 2009; 253(2):281–283

[38] Rahbar H, Parsian S, Lam DL, et al. Can MRI biomarkers at 3 T identify low-risk ductal carcinoma in situ? Clin Imaging. 2016; 40:125–129

[39] Saslow D, Boetes C, Burke W, et al. American Cancer Society Guidelines for Breast Screening with MRI as an Adjunct to Mammography. CA Cancer J Clin. 2007; 57:75–89

[40] Wernli KJ, DeMartini WB, Ichikawa L, et al. Breast Cancer Surveillance Consortium. Patterns of breast magnetic resonance imaging use in community practice. JAMA Intern Med. 2014; 174(1):125–32

[41] Lee CI, Bogart A, Germino JC, et al. Availability of Advanced Breast Imaging at Screening Facilities Serving Vulnerable Populations. J Med Screen. 2015; •; ••:0969141315591616 Epub ahead of print

[42] Kuhl CK, Schrading S, Bieling HB, et al. MRI for diagnosis of pure ductal carcinoma in situ: a prospective observational study. Lancet. 2007; 370(9586):485–492

[43] Warner E, Causer PA, Wong JW, et al. Improvement in DCIS detection rates by MRI over time in a high-risk breast screening study. Breast J. 2011; 17(1):9–17

[44] Niell BL, Gavenonis SC, Motazedi T, et al. Auditing a breast MRI practice: performance measures for screening and diagnostic breast MRI. J Am Coll Radiol. 2014; 11(9):883–889

[45] Kuhl CK, Schrading S, Strobel K, Schild HH, Hilgers RD, Bieling HB. Abbreviated breast magnetic resonance imaging (MRI): first postcontrast subtracted images and maximum-intensity projection-a novel approach to breast cancer screening with MRI. J Clin Oncol. 2014; 32:2304–10

[46] Mango VL, Morris EA, David, , Dershaw D, et al. Abbreviated protocol for breast MRI: are multiple sequences needed for cancer detection? Eur J Radiol. 2015; 84:65–70

[47] Grimm LJ, Soo MS, Yoon S, Kim C, Ghate SV, Johnson KS. Abbreviated screening protocol for breast MRI: a feasibility study. Acad Radiol. 2015; 22(9):1157–1162

[48] Moschetta M, Telegrafo M, Rella L, Stabile , Ianora AA, Angelelli G. Abbreviated Combined MR Protocol: A New Faster Strategy for Characterizing Breast Lesions. Clin Breast Cancer. 2016; 16(3):207–211

[49] Heacock L, Melsaether AN, Heller SL, et al. Evaluation of a known breast cancer using an abbreviated breast MRI protocol: Correlation of imaging characteristics and pathology with lesion detection and conspicuity. Eur J Radiol. 2016; 85 (4):815–823

[50] Harvey SC, Di Carlo PA, Lee B, Obadina E, Sippo D, Mullen L. An Abbreviated Protocol for High-Risk Screening Breast MRI Saves Time and Resources. J Am Coll Radiol. 2016; 13(4):374–380

4 Technical Aspects of Abbreviated Breast Magnetic Resonance Imaging: The Original Approach

Christiane Kuhl

4.1 Introduction

In this chapter, we describe the image acquisition technique used by our group for breast magnetic resonance imaging (MRI), in general, and for abbreviated breast MRI (AB-MRI), in particular, and explain our approach to interpreting AB-MRI studies.

4.2 Technical Aspects of Abbreviated Breast MRI

For abbreviated breast MRI, it is important to choose a pulse sequence protocol that is easy to run, that is reliable and robust, and that yields reproducible results. The results published on the utility of AB-MRI have been achieved with the image acquisition technique described in the following.[1]

We use a four-element surface coil that allows ample access to the breast and thus allows adequate positioning of the breast in the coil. Our current abbreviated protocol consists of three dynamic frames (one pre-, two postcontrast acquisitions), and a quick T2-weighted sequence. Details are given in ▶ Table 4.1.

Any motion of the breast during the acquisitions or between the pre- and the postcontrast acquisition must be meticulously avoided. This is best achieved by usingfixation plates e.g. by Noras Medical Systems, Germany. One should use fixation plates that immobilize the breast (▶ Fig. 4.1) in the slice encoding direction. For axial bilateral imaging, this is the craniocaudal direction; for sagittal imaging, this is the mediolateral direction (▶ Fig. 4.2).

In a screening situation, both breasts must be imaged simultaneously. Irrespective of the available MR methods, this is best achieved in the axial plane. Bilateral imaging in the sagittal plane takes about double the number of sections to cover two breasts compared with axial imaging. Accordingly, for AB-MRI for screening, axial orientation is greatly preferable. Axial bilateral imaging also facilitates the categorization of non–mass-like enhancement because it provides a side-to-side comparison of both breasts.

Regarding the choice of pulse sequence, we use two-dimensional (2D) multislice gradient echo acquisitions. For the selective depiction of enhancing tissue, we prefer not to apply fat suppression, but image subtraction, for several reasons.

First, fat is an important "contrast agent" for breast imaging; it is indeed the only "contrast agent" available for radiographic breast imaging (mammography or for digital breast tomosynthesis [DBT]). In mammography, a cancer is depicted and its margin status can be evaluated only if it is surrounded, at least in part, by fat tissue. The transparent fat tissue provides the contrast that is needed to visualize a cancer's morphologic details. Similarly, MR images that are obtained without fat suppression, that is, with fat signal preserved, provide important architectural information that can be used to characterize enhancing lesions based on their architectural features, or based on the effects they have on the architecture of the adjacent normal fibroglandular tissue (▶ Fig. 4.3; ▶ Fig. 4.4; ▶ Fig. 4.5; ▶ Fig. 4.6; ▶ Fig. 4.7; ▶ Fig. 4.8). The level of information of a precontrast, high-resolution, non–fat-suppressed T1- or T2-weighted turbo spin echo (TSE) image is at least equivalent to that of a set of DBT images (▶ Fig. 4.3d; ▶ Fig. 4.6d; ▶ Fig. 4.7f; ▶ Fig. 4.8c). For instance, fine details of the growth pattern of a lesion with respect to Cooper's ligaments are best evaluated if the fat signal is preserved (▶ Fig. 4.6d; ▶ Fig. 4.7c; ▶ Fig. 4.8c). Moreover, retaining the signal from fat is helpful for further categorization of some enhancing lesions such as fat necrosis (▶ Fig. 4.5). Especially breast radiologists who are used to reading mammograms will greatly appreciate the wealth of architectural information that is available if no fat suppression is used, and will be intuitively able to use this information.

Fat suppression will therefore diminish the diagnostic information that is attainable through MR imaging. Fat signal should not be considered a source of "noise," but it does provide important diagnostic information that can be exploited for image interpretation.[2]

Second, fat is an important contributor to the overall MR signal. Active fat suppression substantially lowers the signal-to-noise ratio (SNR) of a given MR image. This is even more problematic given the fact that breast MRI acquisition protocols need to combine fast and high resolution imaging,

Table 4.1 University of Aachen AB-MRI protocol

Hardware	
Type of magnet	1.5 T Achieva, Philips Medical Systems, Best, the Netherlands
Surface coil	Dedicated multi-element four-channel breast coil by InVivo Medical Devices
Breast immobilization	Fixation plates by Noras Medical Systems, Hoechberg, Germany, with fixation in craniocaudal direction (slice-encoding direction)
Type of contrast agent	Gadobutrol (Gadovist, Bayer Healthcare, Leverkusen, Germany)
Dose of contrast agent	0.1 mmol/kg body weight
Injection protocol	3 mL/s power injection, followed by 30 mL saline flush

Pulse sequence parameters		
	T2 weighted	T1-weighted dynamic series
Pulse sequence type	2D turbo spin echo	2D multi-slice gradient echo (fast field echo [FFE])
TR/TE	3,800 ms/120 ms	around 290 ms[a]/4.6 ms
Flip angle	90 degrees	90 degrees
Turbo factor	18	n.a.
Acceleration	SENSE Factor 2	SENSE Factor 2
Type of fat suppression	None	None
Orientation	Axial	Axial
Position	Exactly matching the position of the dynamic series	Prescribed to cover only the FGT volume, not the fat above and below the breast
Acquisition matrix	at least 512 × 512	at least 512 × 512
Field of view	280–340 mm	280–340 mm
Section thickness	3 mm	3 mm
Number of sections	33	Try to us as few sections as possible to cover the FGT. Usually, 25–31 sections with 3 mm will suffice.
NSA	2	1
Acquisition time	230 s	70 s (per dynamic)[a]
Number of dynamics	n.a.	One precontrast, two postcontrast
Timing of dynamics	n.a.	Inject contrast immediately after completion of precontrast acquisition Avoid any waiting time, avoid talking to patient during contrast injection. Start first postcontrast acquisition after complete injection of contrast agent, i.e., during injection of saline chaser bolus. Avoid any delay between the first and the second postcontrast acquisition.

Abbreviations: AB-MRI, abbreviated magnetic resonance imaging; FGT, fibroglandular tissue; NSA, number of signal averages; TR, repetition time.
[a]Depending on (i.e., increasing with) the number of sections.

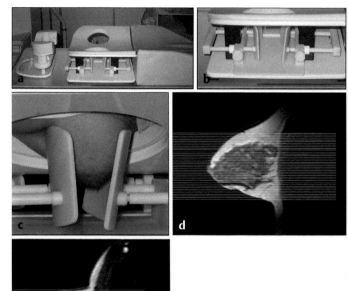

Fig. 4.1 Hardware used. (a) Open breast coil with headrest and breast fixation device in place. The breast coil (in vivo four-channel coil) is open, allowing good access to position the breast. (b) Close-up view of the fixation device. The fixation paddles offer breast compression in craniocaudal direction, which is important for an axial image acquisition (slice-encoding direction). (c) Close-up view with a patient. Note that the breasts are only gently fixated; no forced compression is applied. (d) Sagittal localizer image without breast compression. (e) Sagittal localizer image with breast fixation. Note that less axial sections are needed to cover the fibroglandular tissue.

and are usually acquired by employing parallel imaging. Each of these factors will reduce the resulting image SNR. High resolution imaging implies imaging with very small voxels that contain only a small amount of protons; fast imaging implies imaging with only a single signal average; parallel imaging like SENSE, GRAPPA, or ASSET are associated with another 30% SNR penalty.

Third, active fat suppression takes extra acquisition time; the time needed for active fat suppression may interfere with the temporal resolution (i.e., acquisition speed) and/or the spatial resolution that is achievable. Both, high spatial resolution and fast acquisition techniques per se may already result in borderline (low) SNR of breast MRI; if active fat suppression is added, such protocols may be relatively noisy, thus limiting the detection of subtle enhancing areas.

Fourth, active fat suppression may not work reliably for large-field-of-view (FOV), bilateral breast imaging. Yet for screening, both breasts must be imaged synchronously before and after contrast. This is best achieved by axial imaging with a FOV that is large enough to cover both breasts (not the chest or the upper arm, though). Typical sizes of FOVs will be around 290 to 350 mm. It is challenging to achieve an absolutely homogeneous magnetic field across

such large FOVs, especially since the patient herself will interfere with the field homogeneity. Inaccurate fat suppression is problematic for many reasons; for instance, field inhomogeneities may lead to inadvertent water suppression and thus suppression of cancer signal.

Fifth, active fat suppression leads to the fact that tissues with short T1 relaxation time (e.g. proteinaceous fluid), will exhibit bright signal already before contrast injection. Precontrast bright signal caused by fat suppression means that actively fat suppressed images do also require image subtraction for the selective visualization of enhancing tissue (i.e., tissues that are bright because of contrast-agent-induced T1 shortening, as opposed to tissues that are bright due to short T1 secondary to proteinaceous fluid). Accordingly, actively fat suppressed images do require image subtraction anyway.

For all these reasons, our pulse sequence protocol does not apply active fat suppression, but subtraction. Since we do not use fat suppression, it is essential to adhere to in-phase echo time settings; this is 4.6 ms for 1.5 T and 2.3 ms for imaging at 3.0 T. With regard to field strength, we still prefer 1.5-T imaging over 3.0 T imaging for breast MRI. The theoretical advantage of 3.0 T is its impact on the overall MR signal; compared to 1.5-T imaging,

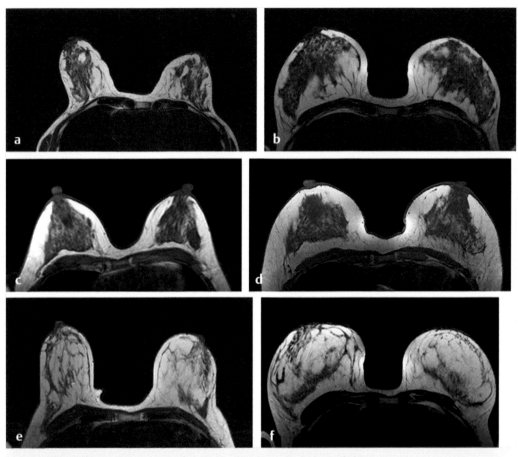

Fig. 4.2 Effects of breast fixation. Several examples of patients who had outside breast magnetic resonance imaging (MRI) studies without breast fixation (column on the left, images [a], [c], and [e]) and received follow-up MRIs in-house (column on the right, images [b], [d], and [f]). In-house MRIs were done with breast fixation in the cranio-caudal direction. Note that the breast fills the field of view better if one uses craniocaudal breast compression for axial bilateral breast MRI. (a) Outside study; T2-weighted turbo spin echo (TSE) image; no breast fixation. (b) Same patient; in-house study: T2-weighted TSE image with breast fixation. (c) Outside study; no breast fixation. Precontrast T1-weighted image with limited spatial resolution. (d) Same in-house study, with high spatial resolution and with breast fixation in craniocaudal direction. (e) Outside study; T2-weighted TSE image; breast fixation in mediolateral direction. (f) Same patient; in-house study with breast fixation in craniocaudal direction.

3.0 T should increase the SNR. However, in our practical experience, these advantages more or less reside in theory. Physical properties associated with 3.0 T imaging such as strong dielectric effects, B1 inhomogeneities leading to variable B1 fields (flip angles achieved) and thus T1 contrast, as well as sensitivity to all sorts of artifacts (pulsation, susceptibility), and the problem of tissue heating (radiofrequency absorption) are all difficult to tackle. There are, of course, methods available to deal with these difficulties, but all of them will be associated with an SNR penalty or reduce image acquisition speed that will, in turn, offset the theoretical SNR advantage. Accordingly, we prefer 1.5-T imaging for breast, and even more so for AB-MRI.[3]

For contrast-enhanced subtracted (non–fat-suppressed) MRI at 1.5 T, we prefer 2D multislice to 3D gradient echo (▶ Fig. 4.9). This is despite the fact that based on MR imaging physics, 2D should have a number of disadvantages compared with 3D, as follows:

- Multislice 2D imaging is associated with a TR (repetition time) that will range between 250 and 300 ms, depending on the number of sections. Compared to 3D gradient echo imaging,

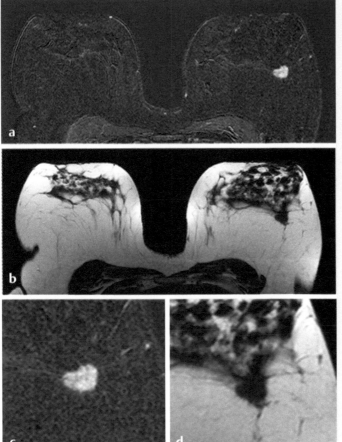

Fig. 4.3 A 67-year-old screening participant, average risk. (**a**) FAST image with a fairly well circumscribed enhancing mass. (**b**) Corresponding non–fat-suppressed T2-weighted turbo spin echo (TSE) image. (**c**) Close-up view of (**a**). (**d**) Close-up view of (**b**). Note that the spiculations and architectural distortions are virtually only visible on the non–fat-suppressed T2-weighted images. Note that cancer exhibits low signal intensity on the non–fat-suppressed T2-weighted TSE images. This is invasive ductal (no special type [NST]) cancer.

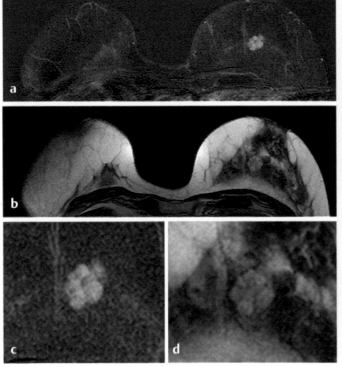

Fig. 4.4 A 63-year-old screening, average risk. (**a**) First postcontrast-subtracted (FAST) image. (**b**) Non–fat-suppressed T2-weighted TSE image. (**c**) Close-up view of (**a**). (**d**) Close-up view of (**b**). Note the roundish, well-circumscribed enhancing mass with internal septations. Mass exhibits high signal on T2-weighted TSE, consistent with fibroadenoma. Note internal septations that are also visible on T2-weighted TSE images. This is a fibroadenoma. BIRADS2, no biopsy recommended. Long-term follow-up confirmed stability of lesion.

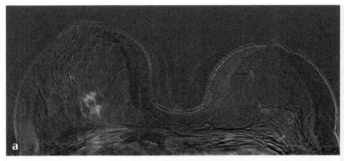

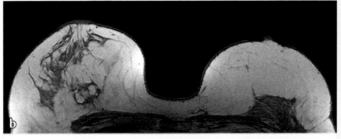

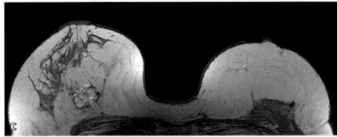

Fig. 4.5 A 70-year-old patient who had undergone mastectomy for breast cancer and breast reconstruction on the left, and reduction mammoplasty on her right, 4 years ago. (a) First postcontrast subtracted (FAST) image. (b) Corresponding non–fat-suppressed, nonsubtracted, precontrast T1-weighted image. (c) Corresponding non–fat-suppressed, nonsubtracted, first postcontrast T1-weighted image. Note the enhancing mass with irregular borders. Based on subtracted imaging, the lesion looks suspicious. Unenhanced, non–fat-suppressed images reveal presence of fat signal inside the lesion (b). This, together with a history of prior major breast surgery, justifies the diagnosis of fat necrosis. No biopsy was taken, but follow-up demonstrated regression of the lesion.

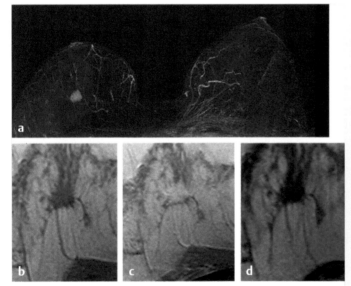

Fig. 4.6 A 59-year-old screening, mild familial risk. (a) Maximum intensity projection (MIP) image. (b) Close-up view, precontrast non–fat-suppressed T1-weighted image. (c) Close-up view, postcontrast non–fat-suppressed T1-weighted image. (d) Close-up view, T2-weighted turbo spin echo (TSE) image. Note an enhancing mass in the right breast that appears fairly well circumscribed on the MIP image. Note that the same mass indeed exhibits spiculations as is visible against the adjacent fat tissue on unenhanced T1-weighted images (b). Note that spicules do enhance (c) and are also visible on non–fat-suppressed T2-weighted TSE images (d). Note that the mass grows perpendicular to Cooper's ligaments as is visible on non–fat-suppressed T1- and T2-weighted images (b–d). Note the enhancing mass appears dark on T2. This was invasive breast cancer no special type (NST).

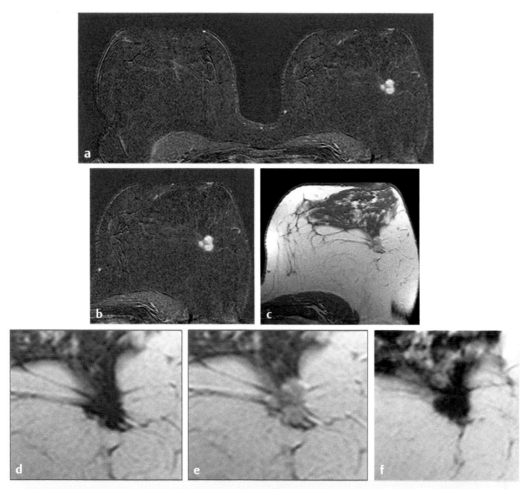

Fig. 4.7 A 56-year-old screening participant. (**a**) First postcontrast subtracted (FAST) image. (**b**) Close-up view of (**a**). (**c**) Corresponding postcontrast non–fat-suppressed T1-weighted non–fat-suppressed image. (**d**) Close-up view of the corresponding precontrast non–fat-suppressed T1-weighted image. (**e**) Close-up view of the corresponding postcontrast non–fat-suppressed T1-weighted image. (**f**) Close-up view of the corresponding T2-weighted turbo spin echo (TSE) image. On the postcontrast subtracted image (**b**), there seems to be a fairly well circumscribed and smoothly bordered mass that even seems to exhibit internal septations. Based on the post contrast subtracted images, fibroadenoma was suspected. Review of the non–fat-suppressed pre- and postcontrast T1-weighted images (**c-e**) as well as the corresponding non–fat-suppressed T2-weighted TSE image (**f**) however reveals that there are no true internal septations, but there are spiculations of the mass and substantial architectural distortions. Moreover, the mass is too dark on T2-weighted TSE to be consistent with fibroadenoma. Biopsy revealed invasive breast cancer, no special type (NST).

this is a relatively long TR, that is, less strong T1 contrast, and thus less sensitivity to contrast-agent-induced effects.

- Moreover, compared to 3D, section thickness of 2D gradient echo acquisitions will be much thicker. Isotropic acquisitions, that is, acquisitions where the section thickness is as small as the pixel dimension in-plane are unattainable with 2D gradient echo. Rather, the pixels or voxels of 2D gradient echo acquisitions will be

greatly "un-isotropic," that is, exhibit a high in-plane resolution, with pixel sizes of 0.5 × 0.5 mm true (noninterpolated) acquisition, but a lower through-plane resolution, with section thickness of about 3.0 mm.

In spite of these theoretical advantages of 3D versus 2D imaging, in clinical practice, for non–fat-saturated contrast enhanced MRI, 2D gradient echo imaging is greatly preferable. In our

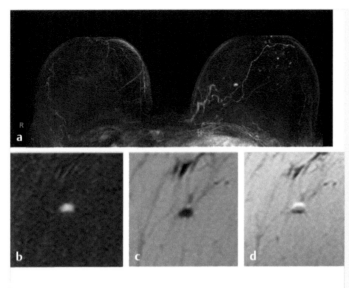

Fig. 4.8 A 57-year-old screening participant. (**a**) maximum intensity projection (MIP) image. (**b**) close-up view, first postcontrast subtracted (FAST) image. (**c**) close-up view, precontrast non–fat-suppressed T1-weighted image. (**d**) close-up view, first postcontrast non–fat-suppressed T1-weighted image. The MIP images demonstrate multiple enhancing foci in the left breast, with one larger focus in the inner quadrant. The FAST image demonstrates an oval, seemingly well-circumscribed enhancing focus with 4 mm in longest diameter. The precontrast, non–fat-suppressed image (**c**) however shows that the lesion exhibits a growth pattern that crosses Cooper's ligaments. Moreover, its growth pattern does not follow the long axis of the breast, because its widest diameter is oriented perpendicular to Cooper's ligaments. This was a small invasive cancer, 4 mm in size.

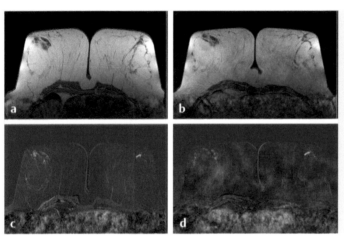

Fig. 4.9 Breast magnetic resonance (MR) with 2D versus 3D gradient echo. (**a**) 2D multislice gradient echo image. (**b**) Same patient as (**a**) examined 2 days later by 3D gradient echo. (**c**) First postcontrast subtracted image of the dynamic series acquired as in (**a**). (**d**) First postcontrast subtracted image of the dynamic series acquired as in (**b**). Note sharp contours of breast in (**a**) (2D) and significant blurring and phase errors in (**b**) (3D). Note crisp contrast in (**c**) (2D), as opposed to "noisy" subtraction in (**d**) (3D).

experiences, this is because of the following: 3D acquisitions are called 3D because phase encoding is used for spatial resolution in all three planes, whereas with 2D, there is a slice-selective excitation. Accordingly, in 3D acquisitions, phase errors can arise in all three dimensions. This can lead to significant image blurring. In 2D pulse sequences, contours of anatomic structures are much sharper. Micromotion during image acquisition will contribute to these contour-blurring effects in 3D acquisitions. To evaluate morphological details of tumor margins or internal architecture, however, all blurring, pulsation artefacts and other types of

image degradation must be meticulously avoided. In our practical experience, this is best achieved with 2D gradient echo acquisitions. One should remember that wherever elsewhere in body and neuro MRI, the focus is on evaluating structure, margins, and architecture for differential diagnosis of lesions, radiologists rely on un-isotropic 2D acquisitions, usually even spin echo based.

It should be noted that the section thickness should not exceed 3 mm because otherwise partial volume averaging effects may in turn interfere with our ability to assess contours of small (≤ 3 mm) enhancing lesions.

In our clinical practice, the fact that 2D gradient echo is associated with longer TRs than 3D gradient echo is indeed advantageous. 2D imaging is a more "conservative" pulse sequence in that it does not aggravate enhancement. It "downplays" enhancement, especially of normal fibroglandular tissue. Since enhancement of benign changes with 2D gradient echo will be less "compelling" or suspicious, we made the experience that the PPV of breast MRI is better with 2D compared with 3D gradient echo imaging—at least if a protocol without fat saturation or fat suppression is employed. Since background enhancement can interfere with the utility of maximum intensity projection (MIP) images, using a "conservative" pulse sequence that does not overemphasize benign background enhancement is of key importance for AB-MRI.

Since enhancement of benign changes are difficult to deal with especially in countries with difficult medicolegal climate, using a "conservative" pulse sequence that does not even exhibit enhancement of benign changes appears particularly advantageous.

If 2D multislice gradient echo is used, it is important to note that one should try to use as few sections as possible. This is because with 2D gradient echo imaging, the TR, and thus the acquisition time, will increase with an increasing number of sections. Our technologists are therefore trained to prescribe the image stack of the dynamic series to exactly cover the volume of the fibroglandular tissue (and not fat tissue above or below the fibroglandular tissue volume). Using fixation plates in the craniocaudal direction serve several purposes here because they reduce the volume of the breast in the craniocaudal direction. With such fixation plates, a usual size breast will be covered by between 25 and 31 sections. A collateral benefit of such reduced number of sections is that fewer sections need to be reviewed by the interpreting radiologist.

4.3 How to Read AB-MRI Screening Studies

If one wishes to start one's own AB-MRI screening service, it is important to collect personal experience with AB-MRI before one uses an abbreviated protocol in clinical practice. For this purpose, one can use educational AB-MRI case series. However, these case series will, with all likelihood, be acquired with a protocol that will differ from one's own pulse sequences. Accordingly, it may be easier

and preferable to train on one's own cases. To do so, just review the respective pulse sequences or part of one's full breast MRI protocol that would belong to one's future abbreviated protocol first, and try to establish a final BIRADS score based on these images. Only thereafter should one review the remaining parts of one's own breast MRI protocol pulse sequences of one's full diagnostic protocol. This will help one to get used to dealing with restricted imaging information on a given lesion.

If one uses dynamic subtracted breast MRI as described here, the abbreviated protocol consists of the following images: (1) the individual pre- and postcontrast T1-weighted gradient echo images; (2) their subtraction that yields the first postcontrast subtracted or FAST images; and (3) their fusion that yields the MIP image(s). Additional T2-weighted TSE images can and should be acquired to help in the classification of enhancing lesions.

The concept of AB-MRI is to use the MIP images for a quick overview and to search for significant enhancement, and then use the individual FAST images, and possibly the T2-weighted images, to characterize enhancement.

Of note, MIP images may not be diagnostically useful in every case. If there is strong background enhancement, this will add up on the resulting MIP image, such that enhancing lesions will be masked. Moreover, if the patient moves, image subtraction can yield bright signal caused by subtraction errors that occur if the position of the pre- and postcontrast images do not exactly match. In such cases, the MIP will appear "bright" and cannot be used for diagnosis, but the individual pre- and postcontrast images need to be reviewed.

If one uses AB-MRI on a broader scale, that is, on women with average risk of breast cancer, it is important not to overcall.[4] One important reason for early high false-positive diagnoses (low positive predictive value) of screening breast MRI studies was the fact that radiologists who read the screening MRI studies were breast imagers who had been trained to read screening mammograms. However, the "reading mindset" needs to be adjusted when it comes to interpreting AB-MRI studies. Mammographic screening provides low-contrast images, and the main task of readers is to search for subtle signs of cancer (subtle architectural distortions; small groups of calcifications). As opposed to this, breast MRI, including AB-MRI, yields high-contrast images. Presence of small enhancing foci or other types of

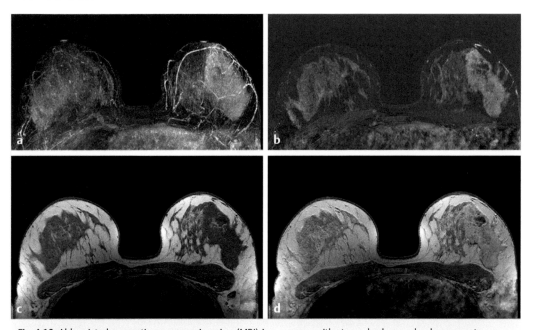

Fig. 4.10 Abbreviated magnetic resonance imaging (MRI) in a woman with strong background enhancement. (**a**) Maximum intensity projection (MIP) image. (**b**) First postcontrast subtracted (FAST) image. (**c**) Precontrast non–fat-suppressed nonsubtracted source image. (**d**) Postcontrast non–fat-suppressed nonsubtracted source image. Note strong background enhancement on the MIP. Still, "dense" segmental enhancement is visible in the left breast. This is confirmed by the FAST image (**b**) and by the nonsubtracted source images (**c, d**).

non–mass-like enhancement is frequently due to normal background enhancement. Readers should call enhancing lesions suspicious only if they observe features that are typical for breast cancer or DCIS. Such features are spiculations, rim enhancement, or growth perpendicular to Cooper's ligaments. Similar principles should apply for the categorization of non–mass-like enhancement; readers should not recommend biopsy unless the MRI features are compelling evidence of DCIS. Features that provide such evidence is either asymmetric, unilateral, clumped enhancement that follows the orientation of the ducts, or "dense," that is coherent enhancement that occupies a segment of the breast (▶ Fig. 4.10). If one obverses a line of enhancement that aligns with a duct, one should make sure that it is ductal, not peri-ductal enhancement.

Readers should be aware of the fact that with AB-MRI, their diagnosis will be far ahead of their time compared with diagnosis of breast cancer based on mammography in the same women. This, together with the fact that MRI tends to depict benign small enhancing foci, tells us that readers should be restrictive with their recommendation to biopsy. Note that there is no need to diagnose DCIS early—only invasive cancer needs an early diagnosis.

If there is enhancement observed on subtracted images (FAST images), one should always review the corresponding nonsubtracted source images to make sure that lesion features observed on subtracted images are not caused by subtraction artifacts.

References

[1] Kuhl CK, Schrading S, Strobel K, Schild HH, Hilgers R-D, Bieling HB. Abbreviated breast magnetic resonance imaging (MRI): first postcontrast subtracted images and maximum-intensity projection-a novel approach to breast cancer screening with MRI. J Clin Oncol. 2014; 32 (22):2304–2310

[2] Kuhl C. The current status of breast MR imaging. Part I. Choice of technique, image interpretation, diagnostic accuracy, and transfer to clinical practice. Radiology. 2007; 244 (2):356–378

[3] Kuhl CK, Kooijman H, Gieseke J, Schild HH. Effect of B1 inhomogeneity on breast MR imaging at 3.0 T. Radiology. 2007; 244(3):929–930

[4] Kuhl CK. Current status of breast MR imaging. Part 2. Clinical applications. Radiology. 2007; 244(3):672–691

5 Techniques for Performing Abbreviated Breast Magnetic Resonance Imaging

R. Edward Hendrick

5.1 Introduction

The goal of abbreviated breast magnetic resonance imaging (MRI) is to maximize sensitivity to breast cancer in a short (< 5-minute) imaging session that screens women for breast cancer.[1,2] The brief imaging duration must include acquisition of a localizing series, a single T1-weighted precontrast series, contrast injection, and acquisition of an single T1-weighted postcontrast series. To perform the entire imaging session in less than 5 minutes, each pre- or postcontrast series should image all breast tissue in 2 minutes or less (▶ Fig. 5.1). Since interpretation of abbreviated MRI is done primarily from the subtracted series (precontrast subtracted from postcontrast series, voxel by voxel) and maximum intensity projection (MIP) reconstructions of the subtracted series, pre- and postcontrast series should be identical and acquired without motion during, or misregistration between, the two series. Modern breast MRI

equipment and fast gradient-echo techniques make this feasible while maintaining the essential features that make breast MRI highly sensitive to breast cancer: high spatial resolution, thin slices, and good signal-to-noise ratios (SNR) over both breasts.

Abbreviated breast MRI was initially proposed and validated by Kuhl et al, using a two-dimensional (2D, or planar) non–fat saturation pre- and postcontrast multislice gradient-echo series pair acquired in a total imaging time of 3 minutes, with breast immobilization.[1] Their results showed that the high sensitivity, specificity, and negative predictive value of a full diagnostic breast MRI protocol could be maintained with an abbreviated MRI protocol that significantly shortens both image acquisition and interpretation times. Subsequent studies have demonstrated that similar high sensitivity to breast cancer can be maintained using three-dimensional (3D, or volume) fat-saturated approaches to abbreviated breast MRI.[3,4,5]

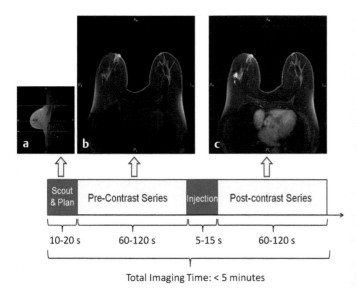

Fig. 5.1 Schematic of abbreviated breast magnetic resonance imaging (MRI) protocol and example images. (a) A sagittal scout view from a three-plane localizer for a 128-slice transaxial acquisition on a 3 Tesla (T) system. The dashed white lines on the scout image indicate the locations of the first, last, and currently displayed slice of a subsequent multiphase T1-weighted series. (b) One of 128 transaxial slices from a 1-minute precontrast acquisition. (c) The corresponding slice from a postcontrast acquisition, displaying a 1.7-cm spiculated invasive ductal carcinoma in the right breast (appearing on the left-hand side of the image). Pre- and postcontrast transaxial 3D acquisitions were identical, with 128 contiguous 1.2-mm thick slices, each acquired with a 487 (phase-encoding, horizontal) × 512 (frequency-encoding, vertical) matrix using a 360 mm × 360 mm field of view, resulting in in-plane pixel sizes of 0.74 mm (phase-encoding) × 0.70 mm (frequency encoding).

Scout & Plan | Pre-Contrast Series | Injection | Post-contrast Series

10-20 s | 60-120 s | 5-15 s | 60-120 s

Total Imaging Time: < 5 minutes

This chapter will discuss the specific equipment and imaging techniques needed to perform abbreviated breast MRI and the technical aspects of breast MRI that can maximize sensitivity in the process. Examples of ideal and less-than-ideal image acquisitions will be presented to illustrate techniques and pitfalls of abbreviated breast MRI. Finally, contrast agents suitable for abbreviated breast MRI and some practical considerations in the delivery of contrast agents will be discussed.

5.2 Essential Equipment Requirements for Abbreviated Breast MRI

Essential equipment requirements for abbreviated breast MRI are identical to those for high-quality diagnostic breast MRI. They include the following:

- A high magnetic field strength (1.5 T or higher), high homogeneity MRI system.
- A dedicated bilateral breast receive or transmit–receive coil with prone patient positioning.
- Strong magnetic field gradients with short gradient rise times.
- A system capable of obtaining good fat suppression over both breasts.

While these equipment requirements have been described in detail elsewhere for breast MRI,[6,7,8] each is described briefly below.

5.2.1 High Magnetic Field Strength, High Homogeneity MRI System

While MRI systems approved by the Food and Drug Administration (FDA) for clinical use have magnetic field strengths ranging from 0.064 up to 3.0 T, systems used for abbreviated MRI should have magnetic field strengths of 1.5 T or higher. There are several reasons for requiring a high-field system. Above about 0.3 T, image SNR per voxel increase approximately linearly with magnetic field strength.[9] Consequently, higher static magnetic field strength (B_0) provides higher SNR per voxel. High SNR per voxel is needed to permit rapid imaging of both breasts with high in-plane spatial resolution and thin slices without losing more subtly enhancing non–mass-like lesions, such as some ductal carcinomas in situ (DCIS).

A second reason for performing breast MRI at high magnetic field strength is to ensure higher static magnetic field homogeneity over the entire imaged volume. High magnetic field homogeneity for breast imaging requires that the static magnetic field strength should remain uniform within about 1 part per million (ppm) across both breasts. At 1.5 T, the resonant frequency of the static magnetic field is about 64 MHz, so uniformity at 1 ppm corresponds to a 64-Hz frequency shift across the entire imaged volume. It is difficult for scanners of magnetic field strengths lower than 1.5 T to maintain a uniform magnetic field at the level of 1 ppm across the volume of both breasts (30–35 cm left to right and posterior to anterior). The main reason for maintaining this high level of magnetic field uniformity is to obtain good fat suppression based on the chemical shift between water and fat over the entire imaged volume, as will be discussed below.

5.2.2 Dedicated Bilateral Breast Coil with Prone Positioning

Dedicated bilateral receive or transmit–receive breast coils have been shown to yield SNR 5 to 10 times that of the body coil (▶ Fig. 5.2). When dedicated breast coils are receive-only coils, the radiofrequency (RF) transmit coils are those built

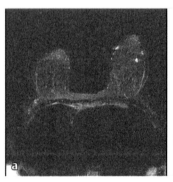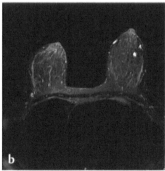

Fig. 5.2 Images of the same slice of the same patient using (**a**) the body coil as the receiver coil and (**b**) a dedicated bilateral breast coil as the receiver coil. Note that smaller vessels visible in (**b**) are obscured in (**a**) due to excessive image noise.

into the scanner bore, the same transmit coils used for whole-body imaging or with other receive-only coils, such as spine coils, abdomen coils, and dedicated coils used for most other anatomical regions. When the breast coil is a transmit–receive coil, the breast coil is designed both to send RF signal into the breasts (to excite measurable signals from hydrogen nuclei) and, a short time later, to measure the signals emitted from breast tissues.

Current breast coils, whether transmit–receive or receive-only coils, have multiple receive channel elements. Bilateral breast coils have between two channels (one channel for each breast) and 18 channels. Multichannel coils record received signals from each channel simultaneously using a different amplifier and analog-to-digital converter for each channel. Like other coils, multichannel breast coils must be matched to the data-handling capabilities of the MR scanner hardware and software to simultaneously record and process multiple channels of data.

When a woman has both breasts, bilateral breast imaging is recommended for a number of reasons.[10] First, comparison of both breasts helps identify focal and asymmetric enhancement patterns that may signal breast cancer (▶ Fig. 5.3). This helps prevent false-positive interpretations due to physiologic enhancement, which tends to be bilaterally symmetric,

especially in premenopausal women and in postmenopausal women on hormone replacement therapy.[11,12] Second, when a breast cancer occurs, there is about a 3 to 5% chance that breast MRI will detect a mammographically occult breast cancer in the contralateral breast,[13,14,15,16,17,18] so it is important to examine both breasts. Third, bilateral breast imaging eliminates some of the artifacts that can occur in unilateral imaging, such as wrap artifacts from the contralateral breast when the field of view (FOV) is set for only a single breast (▶ Fig. 5.4).[6]

Prone positioning in a dedicated bilateral breast coil helps reduce breast motion and respiratory and cardiac pulsation artifacts, without distorting the breasts. The screened woman is supported in the bilateral breast coil at the sternum, lateral chest, and above and below the coil, with breasts pendent within the coils. Providing mild compression to the breasts without deforming them can further minimize breast motion during imaging and prevent misregistration between pre- and postcontrast scans. Any motion between pre- and postcontrast scans or during scanning can cause blurring of images, motion artifacts, and misregistration artifacts in both subtracted images and the MIP images reconstructed from the volume of subtracted images. Mild compression parallel to the

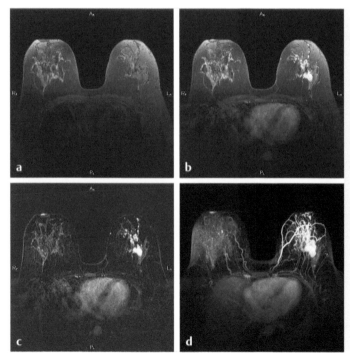

Fig. 5.3 (a) A single precontrast, (b) postcontrast, and (c) subtracted (b minus a) slice in a 3D acquisition in a 41-year-old woman with invasive ductal carcinoma with intraductal component. (a) and (b) were acquired in 3D acquisitions each taking 95 s, with a 340 mm × 340 mm field of view and 448 × 448 matrix, resulting in in-plane pixels of 0.76 mm on a side. Bilateral comparison afforded by transaxial slice acquisition aids differential identification of cancer versus estrogen-related enhancement of normal fibroglandular tissues. (d) Maximum intensity projection (MIP) through all 160 1-mm slices of the subtracted image set, even better revealing the extent of the cancer and the value of bilateral comparison.

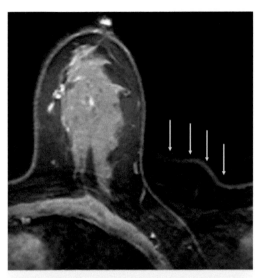

Fig. 5.4 Wrap (or aliasing) artifact of the contralateral breast in a unilateral transaxial acquisition, with phase encoding left to right. Note that the wrap artifact is most apparent outside the imaged breast (*arrows*), but also wraps across and adds structured noise within the imaged breast.

acquisition plane also can help limit the number of slices needed for the screening study. By positioning the patient comfortably and by properly instructing the patient prior to the pre- and postcontrast T1-weighted series pair, rather than after the precontrast scan and just prior to contrast injection, the MR technologist plays an important role in minimizing motion and misregistration. The 3- to 5-minute imaging time of abbreviated breast MRI also should limit patient motion during scanning. Technologists performing either conventional breast MRI or abbreviated breast MRI should be aware of techniques to optimize patient positioning.[19]

5.2.3 Strong Magnetic Field Gradients with Short Gradient Rise Times

Magnetic field gradients are required in each perpendicular direction (x, y, and z) to resolve the volume of tissue within the bore of the scanner into individual voxels. Magnetic gradients are turned on and off quickly many times during a pulse sequence series to select a slice or volume of tissue and to resolve signals from a slice into pixels (in 2D acquisitions) or to resolve

signals from a volume into voxels (in 3D acquisitions).[6] Two parameters characterize the performance of magnetic field gradients: maximum gradient strength, which determines the maximum change in magnetic field over a given distance along the x, y, or z axis, and gradient rise times, which describe the time interval needed to turn a magnetic field gradient from zero to maximum strength. Magnetic gradient strength helps determine how small voxels can be made, while gradient rise times determine how quickly the pulse sequence that resolves signals into pixels or voxels can proceed. The shorter the gradient rise times, the shorter repetition time (TR) and echo time (TE) can be made. This is especially important in 3D gradient-echo imaging for abbreviated breast MRI, because short TRs and TEs are required to produce strongly T1-weighted images in the limited time available for a full 3D series to be obtained (1–2 minutes). Modern MR scanners have maximum gradient strengths of 40 to 50 mT/m and gradient rise times as short as 200 µs, yielding TR values as short as 4 ms and TE values as short as 1 ms. To obtain adequate spatial resolution over both breasts in 1 to 2 minutes per 3D gradient-echo series, TR needs to be less than 6 ms and TE needs to be less than 3 ms.

5.2.4 Good Fat Suppression over Both Breasts

The question of whether fat suppression is advantageous for abbreviated breast MRI is still open. The abbreviated breast MRI proof-of-concept study conducted by Kuhl et al used bilateral 2D gradient-echo imaging without fat suppression.[1] Through discussions with Dr. Kuhl, I have learned that their 2D non–fat-saturated approach is sometimes helpful in confirming the presence of suspicious lesions by seeing lesion margins, and in particular spiculations, in precontrast series as lower signal areas in a background of bright fat. Most dynamic breast MRI exams performed in the United States, on the other hand, employ *3D* gradient-echo imaging *with* fat suppression.[3,4,5,6,8] In this approach, lesion margins and spiculations are typically best seen in postcontrast, subtracted, or MIPs of subtracted series. This chapter's perspective, based on extensive experience with dynamic breast MRI, is that if abbreviated MRI can be shown to be effective using multiplanar 2D gradient-echo imaging acquisitions *without* fat suppression, as it has by Kuhl et al,[1] then it should be at least as effective using appropriate 3D gradient-echo acquisitions *with* fat suppression. The preliminary abbreviated MRI studies using a 3D fat-suppressed approach seem to support this view, at least as far as sensitivity to breast cancer is concerned.[3,4,5] The effect on specificity of performing abbreviated MRI using 3D, fat-suppressed acquisition techniques on a high-risk or intermediate-to-high-risk cohort remains to be seen.

The inclusion of fat suppression in the pre- and postcontrast T1-weighted pair in abbreviated breast MRI improves the conspicuity of enhancing lesions in postcontrast images and reduces confounding background noise and artifacts that can mimic or mask enhancing lesions in subtracted images and MIP images reconstructed from the set of subtracted images (▶ Fig. 5.5). When pre- and postcontrast images are acquired without fat suppression, misregistration of fat between the two series can result in residual fat signals in subtracted and MIP images that can simulate enhancing lesions, especially non–mass-like lesions, leading to false-positive findings. In addition, residual fat signal in subtracted images adds structured noise that can mask detection of subtle non–mass-like lesions characteristic of DCIS, leading, in some cases, to false-negative interpretations.

Unfortunately, there are no clinical studies that compare similar contrast-enhanced breast MRI techniques with and without fat suppression, in either dynamic breast MRI or abbreviated breast MRI. This is due, at least in part, to the necessity in such studies to image each study volunteer twice, once with and once without fat suppression, each time injecting contrast agent.

The next section describes details of the gradient-echo pulse sequence needed to maximize enhancing lesion conspicuity in abbreviated breast MRI.

5.3 Essential Abbreviated Breast MRI Screening Exam

The essential elements of an abbreviated breast MRI exam are as follows:
- Identical pre- and postcontrast T1-weighted gradient-echo acquisitions, each of 1- to 2-minute duration.
- Inclusion of all breast tissue.
- In-plane spatial resolution (pixel size) of 1 mm or less.
- Acquired slice thickness of 3 mm or less.
- Adequately high SNR to detect small (1–2 mm diameter) vessels in MIP reconstructed images.

Each of these essential elements is discussed below.

5.3.1 Identical Pre- and Postcontrast T1-Weighted Gradient-Echo Acquisitions, Each of 1- to 2-Minute Duration

T1-weighting is used in contrast-enhanced breast MRI, as in other clinical applications of gadolinium (Gd) based contrast agents, because Gd-chelates, while shortening both T1 and T2 (or T2* in gradient-echo series), cause a greater change in T1 than in T2 or T2*.[20] Gradient-echo imaging is used

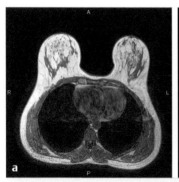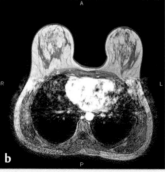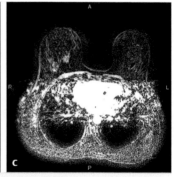

Fig. 5.5 (**a**) Precontrast and (**b**) postcontrast scans acquired without fat saturation and with the body coil as the receiver coil, rather than a dedicated bilateral breast coil. (**c**) The subtracted image (**b** minus **a**) shows artifacts in both breasts due to misregistration of pre- and postcontrast scans, making it difficult to distinguish enhancing lesions from background noise due to misregistration of unsuppressed fat between pre- and postcontrast series.

because it is most efficient in obtaining strong T1-weighting, while permitting high-resolution imaging. Gradient-echo imaging achieves strong T1-weighting by using a short TR value, a very short TE value, and a low flip angle that is matched to the TR value to obtain maximum SNR per unit time or maximum contrast-to-noise ratio (CNR) between lesion and background tissues per unit time.[6] For 3D (volume) acquisitions, signal is acquired from a volume of tissue in position space and phase encoded to separate signal into two perpendicular directions, with frequency encoding separating signal in the third perpendicular direction. This can be thought of as filling a volume of signal data in 3D spatial frequency (or k-) space. A 3D Fourier transform (3DFT) is used to convert the signals collected in 3D k-space into individual voxels in 3D position space. This collection of signal from an entire volume of data, rather than just single planes of data as is done in 2D or planar imaging, adds efficiency to the 3D technique. Extremely short TR values are required in 3D imaging, however, to keep the scan times for the pre- and postcontrast T1-weighted series short, under 2 minutes per series in abbreviated breast MRI. For 3D acquisitions where TR values are extremely short (under 10 ms), gradient-echo flip angles are usually 10 to 15 degrees.[6]

For 3DFT imaging, total acquisition time is $T = (TR)(N_{pe})(N_{acq})(N_{slices})$, where TR is the pulse sequence repetition time, N_{pe} is the number of in-plane phase-encoding steps (to resolve signal into voxels along one in-plane direction, the phase-encoding direction), N_{acq} is the number of times each phase encoding step is repeated (which is almost always set to 1 in 3DFT imaging), and N_{slices} is the number of acquired slices within the 3D volume, which in 3DFT imaging is the number of phase-encoding steps used to separate the 3D volume into a second perpendicular direction, in this case the slice-select direction (▶ Fig. 5.6). Frequency encoding applied during signal acquisition is used to separate the 3D volume into the third perpendicular direction, the frequency-encoding direction, but fortunately does not require an additional time factor to do so. In 2DFT (planar) imaging, N_{slices} is automatically set to 1 in the T_{total} formula, TR and flip angle are increased, and a multislice approach is used. Because in 3D imaging the additional factor, N_{slices}, is large, typically 80 to 160 in breast MRI, very short TR values are needed

in 3DFT imaging to achieve reasonably short total scan times per series. For example, a typical 3D acquisition has $TR = 5$ ms, $N_{pe} = 320$ (the number of matrix elements in the phase-encoding direction), $N_{acq} = 1$, and $N_{slices} = 120$, so $T_{total} = (5 \text{ ms}) (320) (1) (120) = 192,000 \text{ ms} = 192 \text{ s}$, or 3 minutes, 12 s. This is still too long for a single pre- or postcontrast series in abbreviated breast MRI, so additional techniques compatible with 3DFT gradient-echo acquisitions are needed to further shorten acquisition times. These include the use of parallel imaging, partial-Fourier acquisitions, and slice interpolation, each of which is described below.

3DFT (volume) acquisitions have advantages over 2DFT (planar) acquisitions. One is a signal-to-noise advantage because 3DFT acquisitions collect signal from an entire volume of tissue that includes both breasts during each signal measurement, instead of from just a single plane of tissue as occurs in 2DFT imaging. This makes 3DFT acquisitions more efficient, but at the expense of requiring more total scan time (by the factor N_{slices}) to resolve the entire 3D volume into individual voxels. 2DFT acquisitions require resolving only a single preselected plane into individual voxels, using phase encoding to resolve signals in one in-plane direction and frequency encoding to resolve signals in the other perpendicular in-plane direction.

A second advantage of 3DFT acquisitions is that they always subdivide signals in the slice-select direction into contiguous slices with rectangular slice profiles (meaning that all tissues within each slice contribute to the measured signal), while 2DFT imaging typically has small gaps between individual slices and measured signals have Gaussian slice profiles (where signal is predominantly measured from the center of each slice and the signals from slice edges are reduced or lost), as shown in ▶ Fig. 5.7. A third advantage of 3DFT acquisitions is that with thin slices, isotropic voxels (meaning voxels with the same dimension in all three perpendicular directions) or nearly isotropic voxels can be acquired. This in turn enables orthogonal plane or MIP reconstructions of subtracted image data in virtually any orientation without loss (or in the case of nearly isotropic voxels, with only minor loss) of spatial resolution, which can permit better visualization of enhancing lesion margins. 2D or 3D acquisitions with thicker (e.g., 1.5-mm or greater) slices typically

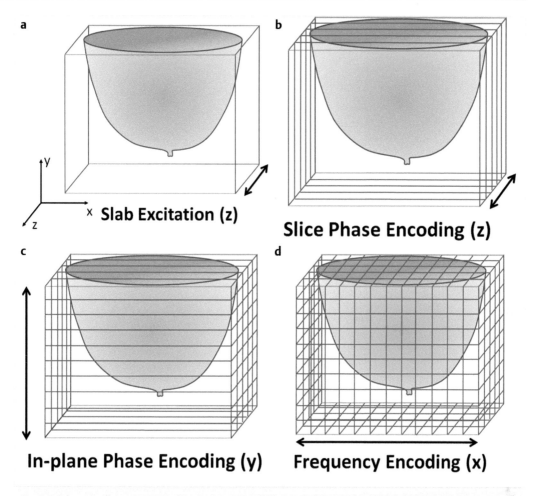

Fig. 5.6 Schematic illustrating 3D (volume) acquisition of slices in the transaxial (*z*-) plane. (**a**) The slice-select gradient (along the *z*-axis for a transaxial acquisition) is turned on to select a slab or volume of tissue to be excited by the radio frequency pulse transmitted into the patient after the patient's breasts are placed as closely as possible to the isocenter of the magnet. (**b**) In a series of pulse sequence repetitions with different amounts of phase encoding applied along the *z*-direction, the excited slab is resolved into slices within the volume. The number of different slices resolved equals the number of slice phase-encoding steps. (**c**) For each slice phase-encoding step, the pulse sequence is repeated with a different in-plane phase-encoding gradient to resolve the volume of tissue into different planes in the in-plane phase-encoding direction, *y*. The number of in-plane phase-encoding views collected for each slice phase encoding equals the number of matrix elements in the *y*-direction. (**d**) During each signal readout, a frequency-encoding gradient is turned on in the third (in this case, *x*-) direction to resolve the volume into different voxels along the third orthogonal (*x*-) direction. The number of different time points at which signal is measured during each signal readout equals the number of matrix elements along the *x*-direction. The total imaging time for a 3D pulse sequence acquisition is $T_{total} = (TR)(N_{pe})(N_{acq})(N_{slices})$, where TR is the gradient-echo pulse sequence repetition time, N_{pe} is the number of in-plane phase-encoding steps (the number of matrix elements in the in-plane phase encoding direction), N_{slices} is the number of slices acquired within the 3D volume, and N_{acq} is the number of times the entire process is repeated, which is usually set to 1 in 3DFT acquisitions.

are limited to reconstruction of MIP image projections along the slice-select direction to avoid the degradation of spatial resolution that occur in other planar or MIP projections, due to slice thickness significantly exceeding in-plane spatial resolution.

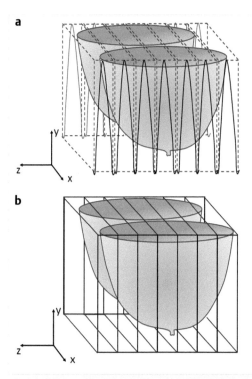

Fig. 5.7 Schematic of the slice profiles in (**a**) 3DFT and (**b**) 2DFT acquisitions. (**a**) In 3D or volume acquisitions, slice profiles are rectangular and slices are always acquired contiguously. As a result, signals are measured uniformly from all tissues in each slice. (**b**) In multislice 2D or planar acquisitions, slice profiles are Gaussian, as shown by the solid black curves, and more signal comes from the center of each slice than from the edges. Often, 2D acquisitions are done with small gaps between slices, shown by the dotted vertical lines, to reduce cross-talk between slices in multislice acquisitions, which further reduces signal measured per slice.

5.3.2 Methods to Speed 3D Gradient-echo Pulse Sequence Acquisitions

Parallel Imaging

To save additional time in either 2D or 3D acquisitions, parallel imaging can be used, assuming the scanner has the software and appropriate breast coils. This is apparent on the technologist scan menu. Many 3D gradient-echo series have parallel imaging options and some permit adjustment of the parallel imaging acceleration factor (AF). For example, if an AF of 2 is selected, scan time will be cut nearly in half for the same coverage, spatial resolution, and slice thickness. Parallel imaging does this by acquiring multiple segments of data simultaneously, speeding the data acquisition process.[21] This acceleration of data collection can occur either in physical space (for instance, one segment of signal data being acquired on the left breast, while the other segment is simultaneously acquired on the right breast) or in k-space, where, for $AF = 2$, every other line of signal data in k-space is sampled and intervening lines of data are interpolated. In either case, the sensitivity profiles of individual receiver coil elements are measured on that patient (which takes a small amount of additional time) to compensate for the simultaneously acquired or missing data and to enable reconstruction of parallel-acquired data into images. One prerequisite to parallel imaging is that the receiver coil must have at least as many channels as the AF. So for an AF of 2, the breast receiver coil must have at least two channels, but could also have a higher number of channels that get combined into two data segments.

In practice, parallel imaging with too high an AF leads to excessive artifacts in the resulting images (▶ Fig. 5.8). Typically, at 1.5 T, AF is not set to be greater than 2, while at 3.0 T, the AF is not set to be greater than 3. Even with $AF = 2$, the time for a full 3DFT acquisition would be reduced from 192 s (in the example of 3DFT image acquisition described above) to 81 to 110 s, a range that would be acceptable for each pre- or postcontrast series in an abbreviated breast MRI exam. The reason that a range of acquisition times is stated for an AF of 2 is that some manufacturers acquire the calibration scan that measures the sensitivity profiles of each coil channel as a separate pulse sequence when parallel imaging is prescribed, while other manufacturers acquire the calibration scan within the parallel imaging sequence itself. In either case, there is a small amount of additional time needed beyond the time estimated by dividing the original series scan time by the AF.

While reducing scan time by a factor nearly equal to the AF, there is an SNR penalty for using parallel imaging. SNR is reduced by a factor equal to the square root of the AF, so for $AF = 2$, SNR is reduced by a factor of 1.41, resulting in an SNR that is approximately 71% of that without using parallel imaging (▶ Fig. 5.8). For $AF = 3$, SNR would be reduced to approximately 58% of that without parallel imaging, although this degree of SNR loss would be compensated by the nearly doubled SNR at 3.0 T compared to 1.5 T, all other acquisition parameters being equal.

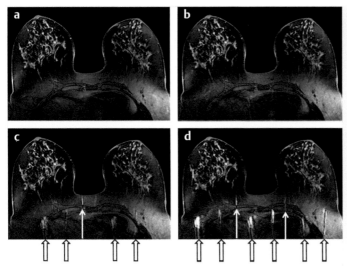

Fig. 5.8 A single slice from 3.0-T transaxial bilateral 3D T1-weighted breast images acquired without (**a**) and with increasing acceleration factors in parallel imaging (**b–d**). In each case, an entire volume was acquired covering both breasts, with identical spatial resolution and breast coverage. (**a**) Without parallel imaging, the 3D volume series took 102 s. (**b**) With *AF* = 2, the 3D series took 57 s. (**c**) With *AF* = 3, the 3D series took 42 s. (**d**) With *AF* = 4, the series took 34 s. Note the increased number and strength of artifacts (pointed out by the black and white arrows) and decreased pixel signal-to-noise ratio as acceleration factor is increased, but without loss of spatial resolution.

Partial-Fourier Acquisitions

A second way to speed image acquisition in either a 2D or a 3D imaging series is partial-Fourier imaging.[6,22] In partial-Fourier imaging, instead of acquiring every phase-encoding view in *k*-space, only a fraction of phase-encoding views (between 0.5 and 1.0, with 1.0 being equivalent to a full dataset acquisition) is acquired; the remaining phase-encoding views (those containing the higher spatial frequency components rather than those comprising the strongest contrast weighting, which occurs at the lower spatial frequency components) are created assuming a symmetry between signal values in positive and negative phase-encoding views (▶ Fig. 5.9). If a partial-Fourier acquisition is done with the phase factor set to 0.75 (or 75%), then three-fourths of the phase-encoding views are measured and one-fourth of the phase-encoding views (half of those in the + or − spatial frequency direction) are assumed based on phase symmetry. Since acquiring different phase-encoding views is the most time-consuming aspect of either a 2D or a 3D acquisition, setting the phase factor to 0.75 shortens the overall acquisition time to 75% of its original duration. SNR is reduced in proportion to the square root of the phase factor, so for a phase factor of 0.75, SNR would be proportional to the square root of 0.75, or to 87% of the SNR without partial-Fourier imaging. Half-Fourier imaging assumes that nearly half of *k*-space is filled by assuming that negative phase signal values are equal to positive phase signal values (with slight oversampling of the low spatial frequency elements near zero along the k_y-axis), resulting in nearly a factor of 2 time savings, with an approximate 40% loss in SNR. In 2D imaging, partial-Fourier imaging can be applied only in the single phase-encoding in-plane direction. In 3D imaging, partial-Fourier techniques can be applied to either the in-plane or the slice-select direction. Application of partial-Fourier techniques in the slice-select direction is the basis of slice interpolation, discussed next.

Slice Interpolation

A third way to speed 3D gradient-echo acquisitions is to use slice interpolation.[6] The principle behind slice interpolation is that a contiguous set of slices equal to about half of those needed is acquired, each with double the slice thickness needed (to cover the full prescribed volume), while intervening slices are interpolated (▶ Fig. 5.10). For example, in a 3D axial series where 16-cm coverage is needed to include all breast tissue in the slice-select or *z*-direction (along the direction of the static magnetic field in a solenoidal magnet) and slices every 1 mm are desired, rather than acquiring 160 1-mm slices, 80 (or 81) 2-mm slices would be acquired and 80 intervening slices would be interpolated from the 81 originally acquired slices. This would result in 160 slices spaced every 1 mm apart. The interpolated slices are constructed pixel by pixel by averaging the signals from the two adjacent pixels, one from each slice, on opposite sides of the interpolated slice.

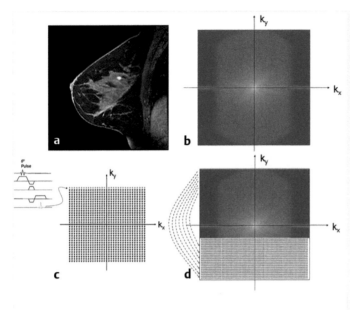

Fig. 5.9 Illustration of partial-Fourier techniques in a 2D image acquisition. (a) A planar image acquired in position space (in x and y). (b) The k-space image corresponding to (a), which shows the signal strength of (a) at each discrete spatial frequency in two dimensions, κ_x and κ_y. (b) is the 2D Fourier transform of image (a). (c) Schematic of a full-Fourier image acquisition where each dot represents acquisition of a pixel value in κ-space. A given row at a fixed κ_y value is filled out during each pulse sequence repetition. Applying a different amount of phase encoding, as is typically done for each pulse sequence repetition, shifts the location of the row vertically, changing the κ_y value. (d) A partial-Fourier acquisition where the upper 5/8ths of the rows are measured, while the lower 3/8th rows are filled in by assuming data are symmetric between $+\kappa_y$ and $-\kappa_y$ values, as shown by the dotted arrows, thus reducing the total image acquisition time to the 5/8ths of that in (c).

When slice interpolation is used, it is important to distinguish between *acquired* slice thickness and *interpolated* slice spacing. It is also important to understand how to prescribe slice interpolation on different scanners. On GE Healthcare scanners, slice interpolation is invoked by prescribing ZIP2 on the scan option menu. In the example above, 80 (or 81) 2-mm slices would be prescribed and acquired, but 160 slices, each spaced 1-mm apart, would be reconstructed in the final 3D volume.

Other manufacturers require the technologist to prescribe slice interpolation differently. For example, in 3D gradient-echo acquisitions on Siemens MRI systems, the slice interpolation factor is set on the pulse sequence menu by setting the "slice resolution," which can be varied between 0.5 (or 50%, which is roughly equivalent to ZIP2 on GE and is essentially half-Fourier techniques applied in the slice-select phase-encoding direction) and 1.0 (or 100%, which means no slice interpolation). The acquired slice thickness is multiplied by this factor to get the interpolated slice spacing. For example, if the pulse sequence is set up to acquire 2-mm thick slices over a range of 16 cm (160 mm) with a "slice resolution" of 0.6 (or 60%), the system will acquire 80 2-mm-thick slices, but will reconstruct and

present the reader with 133 images spaced 1.2-mm apart (2.0 mm × 0.6 = 1.2 mm) covering the same total range in the slice-select direction. One odd feature of the Siemens system, unlike other manufacturers, is that when slice interpolation is selected by the operator, the slice thickness indicated on images (and in the Digital Imaging and Communications in Medicine [DICOM] header in the "slice thickness" location) is the *interpolated* slice spacing, not the *acquired* slice thickness. All other manufacturers report the *acquired* slice thickness in the slice thickness field when slice interpolation is used.

Slice interpolation can only be invoked on 3D acquisitions where, by definition, contiguous slices are acquired. Slice interpolation is completely analogous to applying partial-Fourier techniques in the second phase-encoding direction, the slice-select direction, in 3D acquisitions. Unlike the other techniques mentioned earlier for reducing scan time, slice interpolation has no SNR penalty. In fact, it boosts SNR by acquiring thicker slices—SNR is higher because there are more hydrogen nuclei per voxel in thicker slices—and then interpolating the signal in intervening slices. The only penalty in using slice interpolation is that there is more partial volume effect in acquired slices, since

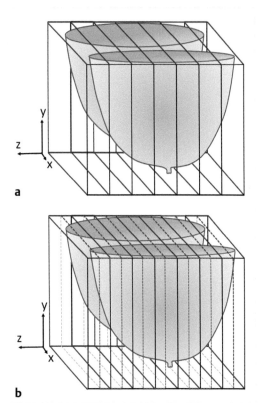

Fig. 5.10 Illustration of slice interpolation. (**a**) Solid lines show the rectangular profiles of acquired contiguous slices in a 3D volume acquisition. (**b**) Dashed lines show the slice profiles of interpolated slices in the z (or slice-select) plane where two adjacent slices are averaged, pixel by pixel in x and y, to determine the signal in each pixel of the interpolated slice. In this example, for N acquired slices, N-1 additional slices are interpolated.

they are thicker. In reconstructed images in orthogonal or angled planes or MIPs, however, slice interpolation is preferable to reducing scan time by merely using thicker slices without interpolation.

Abbreviated breast MRI can make use of one, or any combination of all three, of these time-saving techniques to ensure that the T1-weighted pre- and postcontrast series are each less than 2 minutes in duration.

5.3.3 Inclusion of All Breast Tissues

While inclusion of all breast tissues seems an obvious requirement in any screening exam, it is surprising how frequently the FOV is improperly selected in dynamic breast MRI exams. The goal is to include all breast tissues, to make sure no breast cancers are excluded in the screening exam, while restricting the FOV as much as possible based on body habitus. This is particularly important in the axillae, where breast cancers often occur (▶ Fig. 5.11 a). Technologists sometimes exclude superior breast tissue in an effort to keep scan times reasonable, since more slices in 3D acquisitions means longer scan times, while keeping slice thickness reasonably small to avoid excessive partial volume effects.

On the other hand, sites frequently fail to adjust the FOV and slice range to the body habitus of the woman being examined (▶ Fig. 5.11 b-d). Since pixel size is determined by the FOV and the in-plane matrix in each in-plane direction (the frequency-encoding and phase-encoding matrix) by the formula

Pixel Size (freq) = FOV(freq)/(number of matrix elements in the frequency-encoding direction)

Pixel Size (phase) = FOV(phase)/(number of matrix elements in the phase-encoding direction),

it is important that the FOV be adjusted to each patient to be as small as possible while including all breast tissue.

5.3.4 In-Plane Spatial Resolution (Pixel Size) of 1 mm or Less

Submillimeter in-plane spatial resolution has been shown by Kuhl et al to increase both the positive and negative predictive values of breast MRI compared to lower spatial resolution acquistions.[23] The fine morphologic detail enabled by submillimeter acquisitions yields better visualization of spiculations, irregular lesion margins, and rim enhancement sometimes masked by lower spatial resolution imaging. To achieve submillimeter in-plane spatial resolution, the matrix size in both frequency-encoding and phase-encoding directions should be greater than the FOV in units of mm. For example, when a square 320-mm FOV is used, the acquisition matrix should be 320 × 320 (resulting in 1.00 mm × 1.00 mm pixels) or greater (resulting in submillimeter pixels). Keeping the FOV as small as possible while including all breast tissue improves spatial resolution by minimizing pixel size for a given acquisition matrix size (▶ Fig. 5.12).

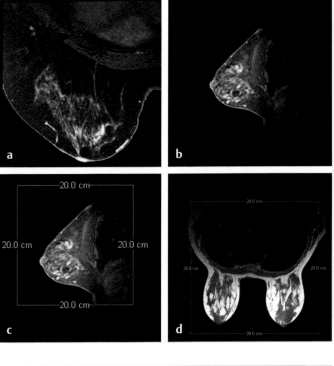

Fig. 5.11 Examples of improperly selected field of view (FOV). (a) Unilateral exam where a 15 cm × 15 cm FOV was selected, leading to exclusion of axillary tissue. (b) Sagittal exam where an excessive 28 cm × 28 cm FOV was used where a 20 cm × 20 cm FOV would have been more appropriate, as shown in (c). (d) Postcontrast transaxial series where an excessive 36 cm × 36 cm FOV was used. A smaller FOV (e.g., 30 cm × 30 cm) would have included all breast tissue and resulted in improved spatial resolution for the same acquisition matrix.

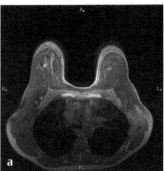
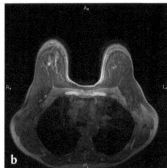

Fig. 5.12 (a) Precontrast and (b) postcontrast transaxial series where an excessive 36 cm × 36 cm field of view (FOV) was used, leading to an excessive pixel size of 1.24 mm in the horizontal (phase-encoding) direction. A smaller FOV (e.g., 29 cm × 29 cm) could have included all breast tissues and resulted in submillimeter pixels, which in turn would have yielded improved detail in enhancing lesion margins.

5.3.5 Acquired Slice Thickness of 3 mm or Less

Slice thickness is important because it sets the limit on the smallest lesions that can be imaged without slice partial volume effects, which decrease lesion contrast. While thicker slices may not impair the conspicuity of high-contrast focal lesions that enhance dramatically, thicker slices can compromise the detection of smaller, low-contrast lesions. To image a lesion of a given diameter without partial volume effects (which would decrease its contrast relative to surrounding tissues), slice thickness of half the lesion's diameter or less should be used. For example, to avoid partial volume effects of a

5-mm enhancing lesion, a slice thickness of 2.5 mm or less should be used (▶ Fig. 5.13 a,b). Limiting slice thickness is particularly important in minimizing partial volume effects on diffuse, non–mass-like enhancing lesions, such as those often occurring in DCIS, which have lower lesion-to-background contrast on postcontrast and subtracted images (▶ Fig. 5.13 c).

Both the in-plane spatial resolution requirement of pixel sizes being 1.0 mm or less and the slice thickness requirement of 3.0 mm or less are specified in the American College of Radiology (ACR) Breast MRI Accreditation Program for dynamic breast MRI and are reasonable quality requirements for abbreviated breast MRI.[24]

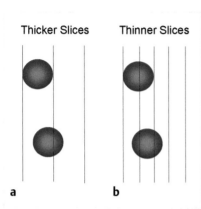

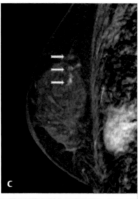

Fig. 5.13 (a) Thicker slices yield higher signal-to-noise ratio per pixel for the same in-plane matrix, but more partial volume effects. (b) Thinner slices reduce partial volume effects and improve lesion conspicuity, especially for lower contrast lesions such as diffusely enhancing ductal carcinoma in situ (DCIS), like that indicated by the arrows in (c) of intermediate grade DCIS with diffuse non–mass-like linear, clumped enhancement in a 48-year-old woman. (Image (c) courtesy of Dr. Robyn Birdwell, MD.)

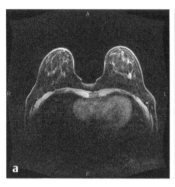

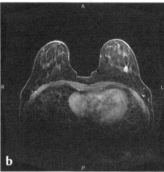

Fig. 5.14 Precontrast (a) and postcontrast (b) images of an enhancing cancer. The two images are windowed identically. The precontrast image in (a) has excessive image noise from an unknown cause, resulting in an unacceptably low signal-to-noise ratio (SNR), while the postcontrast image in (b) has reasonable SNR.

5.3.6 Adequately High SNR to Detect Small (2–3 mm Diameter) Vessels in MIP Reconstructed Images

Being able to see small enhancing vessels (2–3 mm in diameter) on MIP images is an excellent surrogate for the ability to display small enhancing lesions on subtracted or MIP images. Failure to demonstrate relatively small blood vessels on subtracted or MIP images gives the radiologist little confidence that small, subtle enhancing lesions will be well demonstrated, when present.

There are a number of ways that the pre- and postcontrast series in abbreviated breast MRI can fail to detect small vessels and small enhancing lesions. One way is to have technical problems that compromise SNR in either the pre- or postcontrast series (▶ Fig. 5.14). Excess noise in either series will make subtracted images, and MIP images based on subtracted images, excessively noisy, which will mask small vessels and small or diffusely enhancing lesions.

Another way that abbreviated MRI can miss enhancing lesions is to make voxels so small that SNR is compromised. This can occur either by using too high a matrix, so that in-plane pixels size is excessively small, or by using slices that are too thin. Both will compromise SNR to the point that enhancing lesions become difficult to detect (▶ Fig. 5.15). Another way to compromise SNR is to fail to select the breast coil as the receiver coil, which will result in the system defaulting to the body coil as the receiver and lower SNR by a factor of 5 to 10 compared to dedicated breast coils (▶ Fig. 5.2). Lack of fat suppression or poor fat suppression in pre- and postcontrast series and misregistration of pre- and postcontrast images can lead to excessive structured noise in subtracted and MIP images, also leading to inadequate detection of small vessels and enhancing lesions (▶ Fig. 5.16).

▶ Fig. 5.3 shows an example of adequate SNR in pre- and postcontrast images, along with reasonable fat suppression, good image registration, and high (submillimeter) spatial resolution, leading to subtracted and MIP images that show small vessels

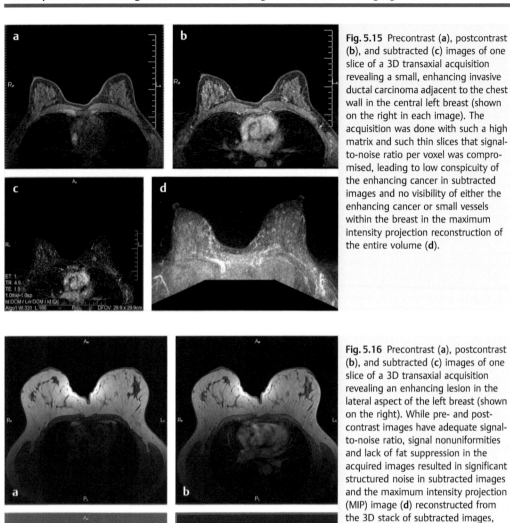

Fig. 5.15 Precontrast (**a**), postcontrast (**b**), and subtracted (**c**) images of one slice of a 3D transaxial acquisition revealing a small, enhancing invasive ductal carcinoma adjacent to the chest wall in the central left breast (shown on the right in each image). The acquisition was done with such a high matrix and such thin slices that signal-to-noise ratio per voxel was compromised, leading to low conspicuity of the enhancing cancer in subtracted images and no visibility of either the enhancing cancer or small vessels within the breast in the maximum intensity projection reconstruction of the entire volume (**d**).

Fig. 5.16 Precontrast (**a**), postcontrast (**b**), and subtracted (**c**) images of one slice of a 3D transaxial acquisition revealing an enhancing lesion in the lateral aspect of the left breast (shown on the right). While pre- and postcontrast images have adequate signal-to-noise ratio, signal nonuniformities and lack of fat suppression in the acquired images resulted in significant structured noise in subtracted images and the maximum intensity projection (MIP) image (**d**) reconstructed from the 3D stack of subtracted images, obscuring the enhancing lesion and all but the largest vessels within the breast in the MIP image.

and enhancing lesions well. ▶ Fig. 5.17 provides an example of adequate SNR and reasonable fat suppression, but borderline spatial resolution, leading to subtracted and MIP images that display strongly enhancing focal lesions well, but lack the visibility of smaller vessels in MIP images that suggest that more subtle, non–mass-like lesions will be well detected in MIP images. The main point is that the ability to detect small vessels in MIP images adds confidence that small or weakly enhancing lesions also will be detected, while consistent lack of small vessels in MIP images suggests that improved acquisition techniques are needed to successfully perform abbreviated breast MRI.

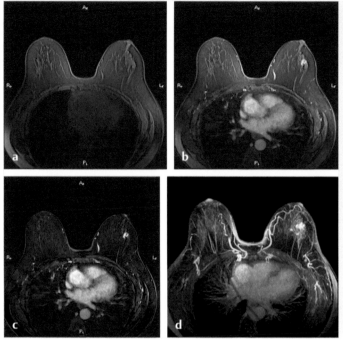

Fig. 5.17 Precontrast (**a**), postcontrast (**b**), and subtracted (**c**) images of one slice of a 3D transaxial acquisition revealing an enhancing lesion in the left breast (shown on the right). Acquisition parameters included fat suppression, with in-plane pixel sizes of 1.03 mm in each direction, resulting in good signal-to-noise ratio, but with lesion margins and vessels slightly less well resolved in subtracted images and the maximum intensity projection image (**d**) than in the case shown in ▶ Fig. 5.3, where submillimeter pixels were used.

5.4 Contrast Agent Considerations

All MRI contrast agents affect tissue signals by shortening T1 (the spin–lattice relaxation time) and T2 (the relevant spin–spin relaxation parameter in a spin-echo series) or T2* (the relevant spin–spin relaxation parameter in a gradient-echo series). Most clinical studies using Gd-based MRI contrast agents perform T1-weighted imaging instead of T2- or T2*-weighted imaging because Gd-based agents have a stronger fractional effect on shortening T1 values than on shortening T2 or T2* values.[20] Another reason is that shorter T1 in T1-weighted imaging causes enhancing lesions to be brighter, making detection easier, while shorter T2 or T2* in T2- or T2*-weighted imaging causes lesions to become darker, making detection more difficult in a background of heterogeneous breast tissue.[6] Consequently, this discussion focuses on the effects of Gd-based contrast agents on T1, although it important to note that any paramagnetic MRI contrast agent shortens both T1 and T2 or T2*.

Relaxivity describes a Gd-based contrast agent's effect on T1 and T2 (or T2*) per molar concentration of contrast agent.[25] The relaxation rate (R1) is the inverse of T1, so the shorter the T1, the larger the R1, and the brighter the enhanced tissue on a T1-weighted sequence. The relaxivity (r1) is the change in R1 per unit concentration of contrast agent. Since T1 is measured in seconds, R1 is measured in inverse seconds and r1 in inverse seconds per millimole per liter of contrast agent (L/(mmol × s)). r1 is determined by measuring R1 at various contrast agent concentrations and calculating the change in R1 for a change in agent concentration (the slope of the plot of R1 vs. Gd-chelate concentration). A higher relaxivity corresponds to a greater ability of an agent to enhance tissues or fluids that take up contrast agent per unit concentration of agent.

Currently, seven general-use extracellular fluid Gd-based agents are used for breast MRI (▶ Table 5.1).[26,27,28,29,30,31,32] Only one, Gadavist, has been FDA approved specifically for breast MRI as an indication.[31] The other extravascular agents shown in ▶ Table 5.1 are approved for central nervous system applications, but are used off-label for breast MRI. The five FDA-approved "conventional" agents (Magnevist, ProHance, Omniscan, OptiMark, and Dotarem) are similar in terms of their concentrations and their relaxivities, which are in the range of 3.6 to 4.7 L/(mmol × s) at 1.5 T. Of this group, gadoterate (Dotarem) was approved most recently, in 2013. This agent has properties similar to the other conventional agents and an r1 relaxivity of 3.6 L/(mmol × s).

Table 5.1 FDA-approved extracellular gadolinium-based contrast agents and their properties

Brand name (Manufacturer), FDA approval date	Generic name	Approved indications	Approved dose	Molarity (M/L)	Protein interaction	r1 relaxivity (L/mmol × s) at 1.5 T in plasma at 37 °C
Magnevist (Bayer Healthcare), 1988	Gadopentetate dimeglumine	CNS, extracranial/ extraspinal tissues, body (excluding heart) in adults and children ≥ 2 y of age	0.1 mmol/ kg	0.5	None	3.9–4.1
ProHance (Bracco), 1992	Gadoteridol	CNS in adults and children > 2 y of age; extracranial/extraspinal tissues in adults	Adults: 0.1 mmol/ kg + 2nd dose of 0.2 mmol/ kg up to 30 min after first dose	0.5	None	4.1
Omniscan (GE Healthcare), 1993	Gadodiamide	CNS, extracranial/ extraspinal tissues, body (excluding heart) in adults and children 2–16 y of age	0.1 mmol/ kg	0.5	None	4.3
OptiMARK (Covidien), 1999	Gadoversetamide	CNS, liver in adults	0.1 mmol/ kg	0.5	None	4.7
MultiHance (Bracco), 2004	Gadobenate dimeglumine	CNS in adults and children > 2 y of age; MRA in adults with known or suspected renal or aor- toiliofemoral occlusive vascular disease	0.1 mmol/ kg	0.5	Weak	6.3–7.9
Gadavist (Bayer Healthcare), 2011	Gadobutrol	CNS in adults and children ≥ 2 y of age; breast for detection and characterization of disease, assessment of local extent of disease, and guidance for localization and biopsy	0.1 mmol/ kg	1	None	5.2
Dotarem (Guerbet), 2013	Gadoterate meglumine	CNS in adults and children ≥ 2 y of age	0.1 mmol/ kg	0.5	None	3.6

Abbreviations: CNS, central nervous system; FDA, Food and Drug Administration.

Gadobenate (MultiHance) and gadobutrol (Gadavist) have been FDA approved since 2004 and 2011, respectively. They differ from the five conventional agents in their physicochemical properties.[30,31,33] All of the general-purpose Gd-based contrast agents are formulated at molar concentrations (or molarities) of 0.5 mol/L (or mmol/mL) except gadobutrol (Gadavist), which is formulated at a molar concentration of 1.0 mol/L or 1.0 mmol/mL. This means that instead of administering 1 mL per 11 lb of body weight, which is the labeled dose of the six other agents, Gadavist should be administered at a labeled dose of 1 mL per 22 lb of body weight (see two paragraphs below for a more detailed explanation).

The relaxivities of these agents reflect the most important clinical differences among them, given that relaxivity is the property most closely related to the signal intensity difference between enhanced lesions and background tissues relative to background noise levels (the CNR of enhancing lesions). Compared to the five conventional agents, gadobutrol (Gadavist) has an r1 relaxivity approximately 20% higher than the other agents (▶ Table 5.1), while gadobenate (MultiHance) has nearly twice the relaxivity of conventional agents, approximately 6 to 8 L/mmol/s at 1.5 T, depending on the methods used to measure relaxivity.[33,34,35] This higher relaxivity has been demonstrated to increase signal-to-background-noise ratios relative to conventional agents by 25 to 35%, an increase similar to that found when going from a single dose to a double dose of a conventional Gd-based contrast agent.[36,37] Importantly, gadobenate (MultiHance) has been shown to provide better diagnostic performance for MRI than the other Gd-based contrast agents in a variety of applications, including central nervous system (CNS),[36,37,38] liver,[39] vasculature,[40,41,42,43,44,45,46] and breast cancer detection.[47,48,49,50,51,52] For this reason, although unproven in this specific application, MultiHance may offer advantages in lesion conspicuity in abbreviated breast MRI, as well.

Some practical issues with regard to contrast agent administration include that all agents should be administered according to the labeled doses, all of which are based on patient body mass and all of which have label recommended doses of 0.1 mmol/kg. The volume of agent to be drawn and administered is slightly more complicated because MRI contrast agents are prepared in two different molar concentrations. Molar concentration is the number of moles of Gd-chelate per liter of solution (mol/L), or molarity. All approved extracellular MRI agents have a molarity of 0.5 mol/L (or millimol per milliliter, mmol/ml) except Gadavist, which has a molarity double that of the other agents, of 1.0 mol/L (or mmol/ml). Therefore, to deliver a labeled dose of 0.1 mmol/kg of body mass, all extracellular MRI contrast agents except Gadavist should be administered based on body mass at a dose of 2 mL per 10 kg or based on body weight, at a dose of 1 mL for each 11 lb, since 1 kg of mass weighs 2.2 lb in Earth's gravity. Gadavist, on the other hand, should be administered at 1 mL/10 kg, which equals 1 mL for each 22 lb of body weight, due to its higher molarity of 1.0 mol/L.

All MR contrast agent administrations should be followed by a flush of at least 20 mL of 0.9% saline solution to ensure that contrast agent is washed out of the tubing and arm and into the woman's major vessels. Since the goal of abbreviated breast MRI is to perform imaging quickly, all administrations of contrast agent and saline flush should be done with a power injector. This is particularly important with higher viscosity agents such as MultiHance.

A practical issue in contrast agent use is that higher relaxivity agents cause greater lesion enhancement for the same labeled dose of contrast agent. If computer-aided display (CAD) systems with color maps are used, it may be necessary to raise the threshold at which color is added to display the presence of rapidly enhancing lesions when a higher relaxivity agent is used. Additionally, because dynamics are not captured in abbreviated breast MRI, there will be no color distinction between rapidly enhancing lesions that have continuous uptake, plateau, or washout. It remains to be seen how breast MRI CAD systems will accommodate abbreviated breast MRI protocols.

In the proof-of-concept study by Kuhl et al, both contrast agent and saline flush were administered at a rate of 3 mL/s.[1] A rate of at least 2 mL/s is advisable to ensure rapid administration of agent and rapid appearance of agent in the postcontrast series. Like conventional breast MRI, the technologist should always check for the presence of contrast agent in the heart and great vessels in postcontrast images to ensure that contrast agent was successfully injected into the patient's circulatory system. If contrast agent is not seen in postcontrast images, the technologist should check the injection site for a hematoma-like bulge of contrast agent in the woman's arm or for a pool of contrast agent on the table under her arm. If this occurs, the woman will need to be re-imaged after appropriate needle placement.

Timing of contrast agent administration relative to pre- and postcontrast image acquisition is particularly important in abbreviated breast MRI since only a single postcontrast series is performed. To proceed as quickly as possible, contrast agent administration should begin immediately after the precontrast series ends. It is advisable for the technologist to prepare the patient for contrast administration prior to starting the precontrast series, not between pre- and postcontrast series, both to minimize the total procedure time and to avoid startling the patient and causing misregistration between pre- and postcontrast image sets.

A final timing consideration is whether the single postcontrast scan should be started just as contrast agent administration begins (without a gap), as contrast administration ends (which would lead to a variable gap of 5–10 s depending on the quantity and rate of administration), or after an additional timing gap to ensure that adequate time has elapsed to maximize detection of enhancing lesions in the single postcontrast series. The proof-of-concept study conducted by Kuhl et al began the postcontrast series after injection of contrast agent at a rate of 3 mL/s and during injection of the saline flush at the same injection rate. Based on a typical body weight of 150 lb (or 68 kg of body mass), a 0.5 molarity agent would require 14 mL of injected agent, while a 1.0 molarity agent (Gadavist) would require 7 mL of injected agent. At a rate of 3 mL/s, this would require about 5 s for injection of the 0.5 molarity agent or 2.5 s for the 1.0 molarity agent, causing a minimum delay between the end of the precontrast and start of the postcontrast series.

Previous work has determined that peak lesion enhancement relative to background parenchymal tissue signal occurs at 1 to 2 minutes after contrast injection for focal lesions and slightly longer than 2 minutes after injection for non–mass-like lesions.[6,7,8,23] Maximum contrast weighting of 3D gradient-echo pulse sequences occurs about one-third of the way into the scan for Siemens systems and about halfway into the scan for most other manufacturers' systems. Maximum contrast weighting occurs midway through most multislice 2D acquisitions, as well. Without adding a time gap between the end of injection and the start of the postcontrast series, a postcontrast series of 1- to 2-minute duration, as recommended for abbreviated breast MRI, will have peak contrast weighting at 20 to 60 s from the start of the sequence. The proof-of-concept study for abbreviated breast MRI had a series scan time of 80 s, with peak contrast weighting occurring about 40 s after the end of contrast injection, resulting in a high sensitivity to breast cancer.[1] This suggests that with manufacturers' current pulse sequences, scans of 80- to 120-s duration per series beginning just after completing rapid injection of contrast agent and bolus should have sufficient enhancing-lesion-to-background contrast to reveal enhancing cancers. It would be optimal in abbreviated MR imaging to have specially designed pulse sequences that place the peak contrast weighting of the pulse sequence (the low spatial frequency acquisitions at or near the center of k-space) at or near the end of the abbreviated pulse sequence, so that maximum contrast weighting would occur at about 90 s after the end of contrast injection. However, this would require MRI manufacturers to provide specialized fast gradient-echo series for abbreviated MRI, customizing peak contrast weighting to be at or near the end of the series, so that the time of peak uptake in most enhancing cancers (about 90 s after end of injection) would occur at the peak contrast weighting of the series, rather than one-third to halfway into the series.

5.5 Open Questions about Abbreviated Breast MRI

Abbreviated breast MRI has been examined in only a few studies, the most complete of which has been conducted by Kuhl et al, at a single institution using 2D multislice gradient-echo imaging without fat saturation and with breast immobilization.[1] Their study showed that their approach to abbreviated breast MRI has the same high sensitivity, high specificity, and high negative predictive value as a full diagnostic breast MRI study. Other more recent studies of abbreviated breast MRI using 3D techniques have focused on sensitivity rather than specificity, recall rates, and negative predictive values,[3,4,5] so the effects of 3D fat-suppressed techniques on these additional important measures of accuracy beyond sensitivity are yet to be determined. It is also yet to be determined whether breast immobilization has a significant effect on the accuracy of abbreviated breast MRI, although these subsequent studies using 3D fat-suppressed techniques without breast immobilization suggest that sensitivity is not reduced significantly with fat suppression without breast immobilization. Another open question is whether the accuracy of abbreviated breast MRI shown by Kuhl et al[1] will be maintained with a broader range of acquiring MRI sites using a variety of acquisition techniques and across a wider range of interpreting physicians.

5.6 Conclusion

Abbreviated breast MRI, like dynamic breast MRI, depends on having adequate SNR, high in-plane spatial resolution to better resolve lesion margins, thin slices to minimize partial volume effects, good breast positioning to minimize patient motion and image misregistration, and consistent contrast agent administration based on body mass or weight, with the additional requirement of completing imaging in less than 5 minutes. Careful attention to the visibility of small vessels in MIP reconstructions of subtracted series gives the radiologist confidence that abbreviated breast MRI will detect not only larger strongly enhancing focal lesions, but also more subtle non–mass-like lesions, providing high sensitivity to breast cancers including in situ cancers.

References

[1] Kuhl CK, Schrading S, Strobel K, Schild HH, Hilgers RD, Bieling HB. Abbreviated breast magnetic resonance imaging (MRI): first postcontrast subtracted images and maximum-intensity projection-a novel approach to breast cancer screening with MRI. J Clin Oncol. 2014; 32(22):2304–2310

[2] Morris EA. Rethinking breast cancer screening: ultra FAST breast magnetic resonance imaging. J Clin Oncol. 2014; 32 (22):2281–2283

[3] Mango VL, Morris EA, David Dershaw D, et al. Abbreviated protocol for breast MRI: are multiple sequences needed for cancer detection? Eur J Radiol. 2015; 84(1):65–70

[4] Grimm LJ, Soo MS, Yoon S, Kim C, Ghate SV, Johnson KS. Abbreviated screening protocol for breast MRI: a feasibility study. Acad Radiol. 2015; 22(9):1157–1162

[5] Harvey SC, Di Carlo PA, Lee B, Obadina E, Sippo D, Mullen L. An abbreviated protocol for high-risk screening breast MRI saves time and resources. J Am Coll Radiol. 2016; 13(4):374–380

[6] Hendrick RE. Breast MRI: Fundamentals and Technical Aspects. New York, NY: Springer; 2008

[7] Kuhl C. The current status of breast MR imaging. Part I. Choice of technique, image interpretation, diagnostic accuracy, and transfer to clinical practice. Radiology. 2007; 244 (2):356–378

[8] Hendrick RE. High-quality breast MRI. Radiol Clin North Am. 2014; 52(3):547–562

[9] Edelstein WA, Glover GH, Hardy CJ, Redington RW. The intrinsic signal-to-noise ratio in NMR imaging. Magn Reson Med. 1986; 3(4):604–618

[10] Friedman PD, Swaminathan SV, Herman K, Kalisher L. Breast MRI: the importance of bilateral imaging. AJR Am J Roentgenol. 2006; 187(2):345–349

[11] Kuhl CK, Bieling HB, Gieseke J, et al. Healthy premenopausal breast parenchyma in dynamic contrast-enhanced MR imaging of the breast: normal contrast medium enhancement and cyclical - phase dependency. Radiology. 1997; 203:137–144

[12] Giess CS, Yeh ED, Raza S, Birdwell RL. Background parenchymal enhancement at breast MR imaging: normal patterns, diagnostic challenges, and potential for false-positive and false-negative interpretation. Radiographics. 2014; 34 (1):234–247

[13] Liberman L, Morris EA, Kim CM, et al. MR imaging findings in the contralateral breast of women with recently diagnosed breast cancer. AJR Am J Roentgenol. 2003; 180(2):333–341

[14] Lee SG, Orel SG, Woo IJ, et al. MR imaging screening of the contralateral breast in patients with newly diagnosed breast cancer: preliminary results. Radiology. 2003; 226(3):773–778

[15] Lehman CD, Blume JD, Thickman D, et al. Added cancer yield of MRI in screening the contralateral breast of women recently diagnosed with breast cancer: results from the International Breast Magnetic Resonance Consortium (IBMC) trial. J Surg Oncol. 2005; 92(1):9–15, discussion 15–16

[16] Slanetz PJ, Edmister WB, Yeh ED, Talele AC, Kopans DB. Occult contralateral breast carcinoma incidentally detected by breast magnetic resonance imaging. Breast J. 2002; 8(3):145–148

[17] Viehweg P, Rotter K, Laniado M, et al. MR imaging of the contralateral breast in patients after breast-conserving therapy. Eur Radiol. 2004; 14(3):402–408

[18] Lehman CD, Gatsonis C, Kuhl CK, et al. ACRIN Trial 6667 Investigators Group. MRI evaluation of the contralateral breast in women with recently diagnosed breast cancer. N Engl J Med. 2007; 356(13):1295–1303

[19] Yeh ED, Georgian-Smith D, Raza S, Bussolari L, Pawlisz-Hoff J, Birdwell RL. Positioning in breast MR imaging to optimize image quality. Radiographics. 2014; 34(1):E1–E17

[20] Hendrick RE, Haacke EM. Basic physics of MR contrast agents and maximization of image contrast. J Magn Reson Imaging. 1993; 3(1):137–148

[21] Glockner JF, Hu HH, Stanley DW, Angelos L, King K. Parallel MR imaging: a user's guide. Radiographics. 2005; 25 (5):1279–1297

[22] Perman WH, Heiberg EV, Herrmann VM. Half-Fourier, three-dimensional technique for dynamic contrast-enhanced MR imaging of both breasts and axillae: initial characterization of breast lesions. Radiology. 1996; 200(1):263–269

[23] Kuhl CK, Schild HH, Morakkabati N. Dynamic bilateral contrast-enhanced MR imaging of the breast: trade-off between spatial and temporal resolution. Radiology. 2005; 236 (3):789–800

[24] American College of Radiology Breast Magnetic Resonance Imaging (MRI) Accreditation Program Requirements. http://www.acr.org/~/media/ACR/Documents/Accreditation/BreastMRI/Requirements.pdf. Accessed August 6, 2015

[25] Tóth É, Helm L, Merback AE. Relaxivity of MRI contrast agents. Top Curr Chem. 2002; 221:61–101

[26] Magnevist® (brand of gadopentetate dimeglumine) Indications and Important Safety Information. Wayne, NJ: Bayer HealthCare Pharmaceuticals. https://www.radiologysolutions.bayer.com/products/mr/contrast/magnevist/. Accessed May 2, 2016

[27] ProHance® (gadoteridol) injection, 279.3 mg/mL [prescribing information]. Princeton, NJ: Bracco Diagnostics Inc. http://www.accessdata.fda.gov/drugsatfda_docs/label/2013/020131s026,021489s003lbl.pdf. Accessed May 2, 2016

[28] Omniscan™ (gadodiamide) injection [prescribing information]. Princeton, NJ: GE Healthcare Inc. http://www.accessdata.fda.gov/drugsatfda_docs/label/2010/020123s037lbl.pdf. Accessed May 2, 2016

[29] OptiMARK® 0.5 mmol/mL (gadoversetamide injection) [prescribing information]. St. Louis, MO: Mallinckrodt Inc. http://www.accessdata.fda.gov/drugsatfda_docs/label/2013/020937s021,020975s022,020976s022lbl.pdf. Accessed May 2, 2016

[30] MultiHance® (gadobenate dimeglumine) injection, 529 mg/mL [prescribing information]. Princeton, NJ; Bracco Diagnostics Inc. http://braccoimaging.com/sites/braccoimaging.com/files/technica_sheet_pdf/MultiHance%20Prescribing%20Information.pdf. Accessed May 2, 2016

[31] Gadavist™ (gadobutrol) injection [prescribing information]. Wayne, NJ: Bayer HealthCare Pharmaceuticals. https://www.radiologysolutions.bayer.com/products/mr/contrast/gadavist/. Accessed May 2, 2016

[32] Dotarem® (gadoteric acid) [product information]. Wayne, NJ: Guerbet; March 2014. https://dailymed.nlm.nih.gov/dailymed/drugInfo.cfm?setid=e2c4a5ac-2df2-4cf4-a2d3-6fbe2-d898ebc. Accessed May 2, 2016

[33] Rohrer M, Bauer H, Mintorovitch J, Requardt M, Weinmann HJ. Comparison of magnetic properties of MRI contrast media

solutions at different magnetic field strengths. Invest Radiol. 2005; 40(11):715–724

[34] de Haën C, Cabrini M, Akhnana L, Ratti D, Calabi L, Gozzini L. Gadobenate dimeglumine 0.5 M solution for injection (Multi-Hance) pharmaceutical formulation and physicochemical properties of a new magnetic resonance imaging contrast medium. J Comput Assist Tomogr. 1999; 23 Suppl 1:S161–S168

[35] Pintaske J, Martirosian P, Graf H, et al. Relaxivity of gadopentetate dimeglumine (Magnevist), gadobutrol (Gadovist), and gadobenate dimeglumine (MultiHance) in human blood plasma at 0.2, 1.5, and 3 Tesla. Invest Radiol. 2006; 41(3):213–221– [erratum in Invest Radiol. 2006;41:859]

[36] Maravilla KR, Maldjian JA, Schmalfuss IM, et al. Contrast enhancement of central nervous system lesions: multicenter intraindividual crossover comparative study of two MR contrast agents. Radiology. 2006; 240(2):389–400

[37] Rowley HA, Scialfa G, Gao PY, et al. Contrast-enhanced MR imaging of brain lesions: a large-scale intraindividual crossover comparison of gadobenate dimeglumine versus gadodiamide. AJNR Am J Neuroradiol. 2008; 29(9):1684–1691

[38] Rumboldt Z, Rowley HA, Steinberg F, et al. Multicenter, double-blind, randomized, intra-individual crossover comparison of gadobenate dimeglumine and gadopentetate dimeglumine in MRI of brain tumors at 3 tesla. J Magn Reson Imaging. 2009; 29(4):760–767

[39] Schneider G, Maas R, Schultze Kool L, et al. Low-dose gadobenate dimeglumine versus standard dose gadopentetate dimeglumine for contrast-enhanced magnetic resonance imaging of the liver: an intra-individual crossover comparison. Invest Radiol. 2003; 38(2):85–94

[40] Knopp MV, Schoenberg SO, Rehm C, et al. Assessment of gadobenate dimeglumine for magnetic resonance angiography: phase I studies. Invest Radiol. 2002; 37(12):706–715

[41] Knopp MV, Giesel FL, von Tengg-Kobligk H, et al. Contrast-enhanced MR angiography of the run-off vasculature: intra-individual comparison of gadobenate dimeglumine with gadopentetate dimeglumine. J Magn Reson Imaging. 2003; 17(6):694–702

[42] Pediconi F, Fraioli F, Catalano C, et al. Gadobenate dimeglumine (Gd-DTPA) vs gadopentetate dimeglumine (Gd-BOPTA) for contrast-enhanced magnetic resonance angiography (MRA): improvement in intravascular signal intensity and contrast to noise ratio. Radiol Med (Torino). 2003; 106(1-2):87–93

[43] Bueltmann E, Erb G, Kirchin MA, Klose U, Naegele T. Intra-individual crossover comparison of gadobenate dimeglumine and gadopentetate dimeglumine for contrast-enhanced magnetic resonance angiography of the supraaortic vessels at 3 Tesla. Invest Radiol. 2008; 43(10):695–702

[44] Attenberger UI, Michaely HJ, Wintersperger BJ, et al. Three-dimensional contrast-enhanced magnetic-resonance angiography of the renal arteries: interindividual comparison of 0.2 mmol/kg gadobutrol at 1.5 T and 0.1 mmol/kg gadobenate dimeglumine at 3.0 T. Eur Radiol. 2008; 18(6):1260–1268

[45] Spampinato MV, Nguyen SA, Rumboldt Z. Comparison of gadobenate dimeglumine and gadodiamide in the evaluation of spinal vascular anatomy with MR angiography. AJNR Am J Neuroradiol. 2010; 31(6):1151–1156

[46] Gerretsen SC, le Maire TF, Miller S, et al. Multicenter, double-blind, randomized, intraindividual crossover comparison of gadobenate dimeglumine and gadopentetate dimeglumine for MR angiography of peripheral arteries. Radiology. 2010; 255(3):988–1000

[47] Pediconi F, Kubik-Huch R, Chilla B, Schwenke C, Kinkel K. Intra-individual randomised comparison of gadobutrol 1.0 M versus gadobenate dimeglumine 0.5 M in patients scheduled for preoperative breast MRI. Eur Radiol. 2013; 23(1):84–92

[48] Martincich L, Faivre-Pierret M, Zechmann CM, et al. Multicenter, double-blind, randomized, intraindividual crossover comparison of gadobenate dimeglumine and gadopentetate dimeglumine for Breast MR imaging (DETECT Trial). Radiology. 2011; 258(2):396–408

[49] Knopp MV, Bourne MW, Sardanelli F, et al. Gadobenate dimeglumine-enhanced MRI of the breast: analysis of dose response and comparison with gadopentetate dimeglumine. AJR Am J Roentgenol. 2003; 181(3):663–676

[50] Pediconi F, Catalano C, Occhiato R, et al. Breast lesion detection and characterization at contrast-enhanced MR mammography: gadobenate dimeglumine versus gadopentetate dimeglumine. Radiology. 2005; 237(1):45–56

[51] Pediconi F, Catalano C, Padula S, et al. Contrast-enhanced MR mammography: improved lesion detection and differentiation with gadobenate dimeglumine. AJR Am J Roentgenol. 2008; 191(5):1339–1346

[52] Sardanelli F, Iozzelli A, Fausto A, Carriero A, Kirchin MA. Gadobenate dimeglumine-enhanced MR imaging breast vascular maps: association between invasive cancer and ipsilateral increased vascularity. Radiology. 2005; 235(3):791–797

6 Abbreviated Breast Magnetic Resonance Imaging Protocols and Clinical Implementation

Gillian M. Newstead

6.1 Introduction

For the past four decades, mammography screening has been the primary imaging method for detection of early breast cancer in the general female population. Mammography screening has been shown to save lives by reducing mortality from breast cancer.[1,2,3,4] However, not every breast cancer is detected by this method, especially when dense breast tissue is evident on mammography. Mammograms are X-ray images of the breast using low doses of radiation and producing two-dimensional projection images. A limitation of this technique is that X-rays may not penetrate dense breast tissue effectively; therefore, these images can be more difficult to read and cancers may be obscured by dense overlapping tissue. Digital breast tomosynthesis (DBT), is a new Food and Drug Administration (FDA) approved mammographic technique that has been shown to increase breast cancer detection at a rate of 1 to 2/1,000 compared to standard full-field digital mammography (FFDM) with fewer recalls and false-positive biopsy recommendations.[5,6,7,8]

Estimates of the false-negative rate for cancers in mammography screening are approximately 10 to 30%.[9] A recent report indicates a mammographic "miss rate" of up to 40,000 to 45,000 breast cancers every year, supporting the need for improved screening methods, especially for women at high risk of developing breast cancer (≥ 20% risk).[10]

During the last few years, evidence concerning the limitations of mammography has prompted many U.S. states to pass national breast density legislation. These laws generally recommend consideration of adjunctive imaging screening methods for women with dense breast tissue. It is estimated that more than 50% of women fall into the dense breast category.[11] Of these adjunctive methods, supplemental whole breast ultrasound screening (WBUS) as an addition to mammography is now the method most commonly used. WBUS has limitations however, principally, high biopsy rates and unwieldy short-term follow-up rates.[12,13] In recent years, studies have shown that compared with mammography and ultrasound, dynamic contrast-enhanced magnetic resonance imaging (DCE-MRI) is more sensitive in detecting breast abnormalities and is an excellent screening tool. MRI uses magnetic fields to produce cross-sectional images of soft-tissue structures. The contrast between normal breast tissue consisting of adipose and fibroglandular structures and breast lesions depends on the mobility and magnetic environment of the hydrogen atoms in the water and fat of these tissues. Gadolinium-based contrast agents (GBCA) are injected intravenously during MRI to improve detection of cancers and other lesions.[14,15,16]

The superior sensitivity of breast MRI compared to other breast imaging techniques has been shown in women with a familial increased risk for breast cancer, and those who are carriers of *BRCA1*, *BRCA2*, or other rare gene mutations.[17,18,19] This evidence has resulted in recommendations from the American College of Radiology (ACR) and the American Cancer Society (ACS) that MRI be used as an adjunct to mammography to improve breast cancer detection in high-risk women.[20,21,22]

There is currently no recommendation either for or against breast MRI screening in women at mild or moderate increased risk of developing breast cancer (15–20%), and the benefits in this population remain unclear. Women with a personal history of breast cancer are at high risk of developing a recurrence or a second breast cancer, and have been shown to benefit from MRI surveillance, with more cancers detected on follow-up MRI when compared to mammography.[23] Although annual mammography is generally recommended following treatment of women with breast cancer, MRI is often added to the surveillance regimen when the patient's age, imaging features cancer histology, and genetic profile are taken into account.

Breast density has been shown to be an independent risk factor for breast cancer. A meta-analysis in 2006 showed that women with dense breasts had a fourfold to fivefold increased risk compared with other women.[24] Breast biopsies performed for diagnosis of mammographic or ultrasound abnormalities may detect atypical hyperplasia, lobular carcinoma in situ, and other high-risk lesions, in approximately 10% of benign biopsies.[25] Studies have shown that the lifetime risk of breast cancer in women with prior diagnosis of a high-risk lesion is about 30% when followed for 25 years,[26,27,28] and additional MRI surveillance is often recommended in these women as well.[29,30]

The sensitivity of breast MRI has been shown to be substantially higher than mammography even for women at average breast cancer risk. A major criticism of MRI screening points to low specificity and a high rate of follow-up examinations and biopsies. However, a recent study of MR examinations in average risk women showed a 33% (18/54) positive predictive value (PPV) at MRI-recommended biopsy, a rate which fares favorably to the accepted PPV rate for other modalities such as mammography and ultrasound.[31] Early studies involving interpretations of an abbreviated MRI (AB-MR) protocol have shown equivalent sensitivity for cancer detection when compared to a full standard MRI, with only minimal decrease in specificity,[32,33] and this growing evidence suggests a benefit for the expanded use of breast MRI for screening of a larger section of the female population, and poses an exciting challenge. The challenge will be to develop streamlined, efficient, workflow to allow for rapid screening at a lower cost. This effort will evoke memories of the early days of screening mammography when new methods were developed to introduce screening into radiology practices for the first time.[34] The excitement will come from our ability to improve the detection of an increased numbers of small cancers, most of them node negative, for the benefit of a much larger population of women. Key to this process will be a faster MRI protocol, efficient throughput, and advanced training for radiologists in the interpretation of MRI screening studies.

6.2 Standard Dynamic Contrast-Enhanced Magnetic Resonance Imaging Protocols

The basic MRI acquisition protocol for breast MRI has not changed greatly over the past two decades. Principally, the standard of care has included a precontrast T2-weighted acquisition followed by a dynamic contrast-enhanced (DCE-MRI) sequence, consisting of a series of T1-weighted acquisitions before and for approximately 5 to 7 minutes after the intravenous administration of contrast media. The contrast agents used clinically are gadolinium based (GBCM). The effect of gadolinium reduces the T1 in its microenvironment, increasing its signal in a T1-weighted acquisition; therefore, regions or lesions with increased blood flow and

permeability such as cancers will accumulate contrast media to a greater extent than the surrounding tissue, resulting in higher signal increase. Lesion conspicuity therefore increases after the injection of contrast media and is highlighted on subtraction images (postcontrast minus baseline images). The temporal resolution of MR acquisition protocols in the United States has generally remained between 90 to 120 seconds in most practices, with a maximum resolution of 240 seconds allowed in the ACR Accreditation Program.[35] The Breast Magnetic Resonance Imaging Accreditation Program, sponsored by the ACR, requires both a T2-weighted (bright fluid) series and a multiphase T1-weighted series. The dynamic series must include a precontrast T1-weighted series, an early-phase (first) postcontrast T1-weighted series to be completed within 4 minutes of contrast injection, and a late-phase T1-weighted series with features matching the precontrast T1-weighted series. Measures of the rate of uptake and washout of contrast media within breast lesions contain diagnostically useful information. The shape of the signal intensity versus time curve (or signal time-course or kinetic curve) has shown to be useful in the classification of enhancing lesions.[36] Lesions with a fast uptake of contrast followed by a washout phase are more likely to be malignant, while lesions with a slow but persistent uptake are more likely benign. Discrete thresholds are used to classify two parts of the kinetic curve: the initial uptake and the delayed phase. Computer-aided diagnostic (CAD) systems can improve physician interpretation workflow by organizing and presenting large image datasets for interpretation, and by providing automatic analysis of the kinetic characteristics of enhancing lesions. Advanced computer displays can expedite kinetic characteristics by placing colored overlays on voxels within an enhancing lesion, thereby demonstrating the kinetics of the delayed phase of lesion enhancement as washout, plateau, or persistent, and the initial rise as slow, medium, or rapid. Additional provision of both time intensity curves and angiomaps allows a convenient and efficient way for radiologists to assess lesion enhancement kinetics. Microvascular density is a key factor in determining the initial rate of contrast media uptake and the heterogeneity within tumor enhancement.[37] There is some overlap between the kinetic assessment of benign and malignant lesions at MRI; therefore, the kinetic classification alone, while valuable (diagnostic accuracy 86%), is not sufficient for accurate diagnosis, and combined analysis of lesion morphology and kinetic characteristics is necessary.

The accuracy of MR interpretation may be affected by the variable enhancement of normal breast tissue, which usually enhances slowly initially, generates a persistent kinetic curve, and is referred to as background parenchymal enhancement (BPE). The hormonal response of breast tissue in premenopausal women varies during the menstrual cycle. Marked BPE can limit the sensitivity of the examination[38,39] because differentiation of enhancing abnormalities from BPE may present a diagnostic challenge.[40] For this reason, it is recommended that premenopausal women should ideally be scanned during the second week of the menstrual cycle and week 4 should be avoided if at all possible.[41]

At the University of Chicago (UC), the current routine clinical breast MRI protocol at field strengths 1.5 and 3.0 T includes a T2-weighted, non–fat-suppressed axial sequence followed by a T1-weighted fat-suppressed axial dynamic series, with images acquired before and after intravenous administration of contrast media. At 3.0 T, five postcontrast acquisitions at a temporal resolution of approximately 60 seconds and spatial resolution of 0.8 × 0.8 × 0.8 cm are obtained for both the T2-weighted and the T1-weighted series. The images from both acquired series are isotropic, matched spatially, and allow multiplanar formatting of both the T2-weighted and the T1-weighted sequences with identical spatial resolution in all planes as shown in ▶ Fig. 6.1.

6.3 Semiquantitative Analysis of Dynamic Contrast-Enhanced Magnetic Resonance Imaging

Routine interpretation of DCE-MRI studies is based on signal intensity and how it changes with time after the injection of contrast media. The semiquantitative kinetic analysis, as shown in the previously described standard protocol, has the advantage of being relatively simple to implement in routine clinical practice. Intrinsic lesion characteristics, acquisition parameters, and concentration all play a role in signal enhancement. While the discrete categorization of lesion kinetics has been shown to be diagnostically useful, previous work by Jansen et al[42] found that the descriptors of curve shape vary significantly between different scanners and acquisition parameters in malignant lesions. Semiquantitative methods are mostly focused on the analysis of the lesion kinetic curve. Therefore, diagnostic tools such as the standard signal intensity time course curves may be difficult to apply across different sites, because their

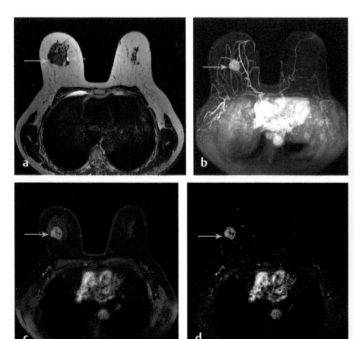

Fig. 6.1 A 56-year-old woman presents with a newly diagnosed invasive duct cancer grade 2, in the right breast at 12 o'clock. A standard breast MRI protocol is shown at 3 Tesla (T). (a) Shows an isointense mass on the T2-weighted (T2w) non–fat-saturated axial precontrast image (*long arrow*) with a small medial adjacent cyst (*short arrow*). The invasive cancer is well seen on the axial T1w maximum intensity projection image (MIP) at 1 minute postcontrast injection, (b) (*arrow*), and also the axial source and subtraction images at 1 minute postcontrast, (c) and (d) (*arrows*). It should be noted that both the T2w and the T1w images are isotropic allowing optimal multiplanar reformatting.

performance will depend on the particular thresholds chosen for each scanner. A study by Pineda et al found that semiquantitative descriptors of curve shape can vary significantly in repeated scans of the same patients at different field strengths.[43]

Direct measurement of the signal increase or percent signal enhancement in DCE-MRI is not equivalent to measuring the concentration of contrast media in tissues. Conversion from signal intensity to concentration of contrast media is necessary for pharmacokinetic (PK) analysis of DCE-MRI data. The goal of PK analysis (also referred to as tracer kinetic modeling) is to estimate quantitative parameters that describe blood flow, capillary leakage, and related physiological parameters. The most widely used model in PK analysis of breast lesions is the two-compartment model (TCM) and the formalism first proposed by Kety and applied to DCE-MRI by Tofts.[44,45] This model assumes two compartments where contrast media is distributed, the blood plasma and the extravascular extracellular space (EES or v_e). The exchange of contrast media between the blood plasma compartment and the EES is described by the transfer rate constant (K_{trans}). The redistribution rate constant, k_{ep}, is defined as the ratio of K_{trans} to v_e and determines the transfer of contrast media from the lesion back into the plasma. K_{trans} is related to the blood flow in the capillary, its permeability, and surface area. Because permeability is greater in tumors due to the fenestration of the vasculature feeding them, K_{trans} may be a diagnostically useful quantity. Despite these limitations, studies have shown significant correlation between semiquantitative and quantitative methods. Measurements such as the initial area under the time course contrast curve (iAUC), have been shown to correlate with standard PK parameters (K_{trans}, k_{ep}, and v_e), suggesting that it may be possible to identify semiquantitative parameters from routine DCE-MRI acquisitions that reflect directly the biology of enhancing lesions.[46] Further research will be necessary to determine whether semiquantitative parameters can be accurately correlated with PK parameters in clinical practice, and whether these parameters factors can be standardized across different MR platforms and acquisition protocols.

6.4 Quantitative Analysis of Dynamic Contrast-Enhanced Magnetic Resonance Imaging

Quantitative analysis of DCE-MRI, such as PK modeling, has been shown to yield useful prognostic information and has the potential to increase the diagnostic accuracy of DCE-MRI by probing directly the physiological properties of tumors.[47] Calculations of contrast media concentration within an enhancing lesion provide important physiologic information and added diagnostic value. In order to incorporate analysis based on lesion concentration of contrast media into clinical practice, measures of the relaxivity of the contrast agent, the arterial input function,[48,49,50,51] the B1 field of the transmitter,[52,53,54] the native or baseline T1 of an identified lesion,[46] and the shortened postcontrast T1 at each time point in the DCE sequence are required.[45,49,50,51,52,55,56]

Quantitative analysis, starting with the calculation of the actual concentration of contrast in enhancing lesions, has the potential to standardize DCE-MRI for multicenter and longitudinal studies, and to produce PK parameters that relate directly to intrinsic physiology and biology. Ongoing research into quantitative analysis of DCE-MRI methods could improve discrimination between benign and malignant lesions, and also produce an imaging biomarker with prognostic value and the potential to guide therapy.[57]

6.5 Abbreviated Magnetic Resonance Protocol: Abbreviated Breast Magnetic Resonance Imaging

In the first study of its kind, Kuhl et al recently reported on the results of an abbreviated MRI protocol and showed that a shorter (3-minute) MRI was comparable to the accepted standard of 21-minute study when screening for cancer.[58] Although this protocol is likely not sufficient for a complete diagnostic examination, in the screening setting this study showed a high detection rate without a corresponding high false-positive rate, an indication of an excellent high-quality screening test. Of the 11 cancers diagnosed in 603 women in this study, most were intermediate or high nuclear grade with a median size of 8.4 mm, and all malignancies were node negative. These excellent results have prompted other researchers to consider further development of shorter MR imaging protocols for screening. Potential additional benefits could include better patient tolerance for a shorter MR examination and reduced costs, resulting in improved screening not only for high-risk women, but also for women at mild to moderate increased risk as well.

6.6 Abbreviated Breast Magnetic Resonance Imaging: Adapted Standard Protocol

In addition to the AB-MR protocol devised by Kuhl et al,[58] any standard diagnostic protocol currently used in clinical practice can be shortened to accomplish an effective abbreviated protocol for screening. Generally, a T2-weighted sequence and a dynamic contrast-enhanced sequence with one or two postcontrast series will suffice, achieving a total acquisition time of 10 minutes or less. The MRI study should fulfill the following requirements: standardized contrast administration based on kilogram weight using a power injector, total scan time of less than 10 minutes (including localizer), one precontrast and one or two postcontrast gradient echo (GRE) fat-suppressed axial acquisitions, with in-plane resolution of 1 mm or less, slice thickness of 3 mm of less. An additional axial T2-weighted sequence with in-plane resolution matching the GRE sequences and 3 mm or less slice thickness is useful for improved specificity. Technical parameters for an abbreviated breast (AB-MR) protocol, adapted from a standard clinical protocol at UC, for both 1.5- and 3.0-T magnets, are shown in ▶ Table 6.1 and ▶ Table 6.2, respectively.

6.7 Abbreviated Breast Magnetic Resonance Imaging: Innovative Protocols

New protocols, referred to as "ultrafast imaging," are currently under development aimed toward imaging and sampling early kinetics at a faster rate, 4 to 8 seconds (s) per time point for a bilateral scan. DCE-MRI examinations at UC include a high temporal resolution, lower spatial resolution acquisition during the first minute following contrast injection, followed by a standard, higher spatial resolution image acquisition, achieving a total acquisition time of 3 minutes for dynamic scans. Early work by this group[59] and others[60] demonstrated that this type of early acquisition often increases lesion conspicuity relative to a standard clinical protocol. Lesion conspicuity in ultrafast (UF) images is often greatest within the first 30 seconds after contrast media injection, when parenchymal enhancement is minimal, even when marked BPE is found on later images.[43,61] UF DCE-MRI methods allow measurement of the rate of lesion enhancement with respect to time, of initial arterial enhancement in the breast,[62] rather than time of injection, thus reducing dependence on global variables such as cardiac output.

An example of UF DCE-MRI is shown in ▶ Fig. 6.2. The patient presented with known invasive duct carcinoma in the right breast showing maximum intensity projections (MIPs) generated from bilateral subtraction images acquired with a 6.6-second temporal resolution. Each image is labeled with the time of postcontrast injection. Arteries, including those feeding the lesion in the right breast, enhance a few seconds before the cancer. The arteries feeding the lesion and draining veins are easily detectable in early images but less visible in later images. The cancer enhances before normal parenchyma, which is a considerable advantage when marked BPE is present on later images.

UF DCE-MRI allows new approaches to quantitative data analysis, including measurements of the initial rate of lesion enhancement. Time of arrival (TOA) of the contrast bolus can be accurately measured relative to the initial enhancement in the artery. This potentially powerful approach can correct for variations in contrast media injection speed and cardiac output, allowing for more standardized measurements. ▶ Fig. 6.3 illustrates this approach. The images show the TOA of the contrast bolus in each pixel relative to the initial enhancement in arteries. The invasive cancer enhances almost simultaneously with the arteries; thus, it is indicated in red—since TOA is close to "0." However, the complex sclerosing lesion (radial scar) enhances much later (▶ Fig. 6.3).

UF imaging may also have other advantages. Measurement of small, early enhancement allows simplified and more accurate measurements of the arterial input function and K_{trans}. With adequate temporal resolution, propagation of the contrast media bolus through arteries feeding lesions and the draining veins can be imaged, and this may provide additional diagnostically useful information. Preliminary results suggest that there are significant differences between benign and malignant lesions in parameters that describe contrast media uptake kinetics in the first minute postinjection of contrast media.

UF bilateral images acquired at UC use standard Cartesian k-space sampling. This is different

Table 6.1 AB-MR: adapted standard protocol at 1.5 T (Phillips)

1. VISTA (non–fat-suppressed T2 weighted)

1. DCE-MRI (fat-suppressed T1 weighted): precontrast mask, followed by standard DCE-MRI for two postcontrast acquisitions

Parameters

	VISTA	DCE-MRI
Geometry	3D axial	3D axial
FOV (mm)	320–400	320–400
Spatial resolution/interpolated (mm)	0.8/0.8	0.8/0.7
Slice thickness/interpolated (mm)	2.0/1.0	2.0/1.0
Number of slices	200	175
Slice oversample	default	1.0
Slice gap (mm)	N/A	N/A
SENSE acceleration	3 × 2	2.5 × 2.0
TR (ms)	2,000	5.5
TE (ms)	368	2.7
Flip angle (degrees)	90	12
Fast imaging mode	TSE	TFE
Fast imaging factor	120	44
Fat suppression	None	SPAIR
Partial Fourier imaging	No	No
k-space sampling	Cartesian	Cartesian
Number of averages	1	1
Duration (m:s)	2:32	5:24
Temporal resolution (m:s)	N/A	0:54
b values (s/mm²)	N/A	N/A

Abbreviations: AB-MR, abbreviated breast magnetic resonance imaging; DCE-MRI, dynamic contrast-enhanced MRI; FOV, field of view; N/A, not available; SPAIR, short scar periareolar inferior pedicle reduction; TE, echo time; TFE, turbo field echo; TR, repetition time; TSE, turbo spin echo.
Note: Parameters for VISTA and DCE-MRI are standard clinical parameters, so there is no special consideration to their selection beyond optimization for image quality in given time.

from the "view sharing" methods that are often used to image at high temporal resolution in DCE-MRI clinical protocols. Keyhole approaches and other "view sharing" methods like "TRICKS" and "TWIST" typically involve scanning the center of k-space at relatively high temporal resolution, and the outer portions of k-space at much lower temporal resolution.[63,64,65] Each image in the dynamic series is produced from data from different parts of k-space scanned at different times. This results in high-quality images, but it is difficult to perform quantitative analysis of data acquired with these sequences. Problems arise when data are analyzed to determine which features are enhancing at what strength and at what rate, particularly in the case of small features (e.g., lesions) with sharp and irregular edges. The information from the initial 10 seconds after uptake initiation is combined with information from other time periods, and

Table 6.2 AB-MR: adapted standard protocol 3.0-T scanner (Phillips)

1. VISTA (non–fat-suppressed T2 weighted)

1. DCE-MRI (fat-suppressed T1 weighted): precontrast mask, followed by standard DCE-MRI for two postcontrast acquisitions

Parameters

	VISTA	DCE-MRI
Geometry	3D axial	3D axial
FOV (mm)	320–400	320–400
Spatial resolution/interpolated (mm)	0.8/0.65	0.8/0.6
Slice thickness/interpolated (mm)	1.6/0.8	1.6/0.8
Number of slices	250	250
Slice oversample	1.33	1.0
Slice gap (mm)	N/A	N/A
SENSE acceleration	3 × 2	2.5 × 2.0
TR (ms)	2000	4.8
TE (ms)	221	2.4
Flip angle (degrees)	90	10
Fast imaging mode	TSE	TFE
Fast imaging factor	120	27
Fat suppression	None	SPAIR
Partial Fourier imaging	No	0.85 × 1.0
k-space sampling	Cartesian	Cartesian
Number of averages	1	1
Duration (m:s)	3:44	2:13
Temporal resolution (m:s)	N/A	1:02
b values (s/mm^2)	N/A	N/A

Abbreviations: AB-MR, abbreviated breast magnetic resonance imaging; DCE-MRI, dynamic contrast-enhanced MRI; FOV, field of view; N/A, not available; SPAIR; short scar periareolar inferior pedicle reduction; TE, echo time; TFE, turbo field echo; TR, repetition time; TSE, turbo spin echo.
Note: Parameters for VISTA and DCE-MRI are standard clinical parameters, so there is no special consideration to their selection beyond optimization for image quality in given time.

the diagnostic utility is thus diluted. For example, if a narrow blood vessel, the rim of a cancer, or spiculations on a suspicious lesion appear to enhance rapidly, it is difficult to determine the true rate of enhancement.[61] Compressed sensing methods have similar problems and produce artifacts.[66,67,68]

Over the past year, at both 1.5 and 3.0 T, we have incorporated a UF sequence with 6- to 9-second temporal resolution into the dynamic acquisition portion of our standard diagnostic clinical DCE-MRI protocol and our AB-MR screening protocol at UC. Prerequisites for the AB-MR protocol include standardized contrast administration based on kilogram weight using a power injector, and total imaging time of less than 10 minutes (including localizer). Two precontrast and eight postcontrast 6- to 9-second UF acquisitions are obtained followed by one standard 70-second GRE axial acquisition. In this protocol, the UF slice thickness

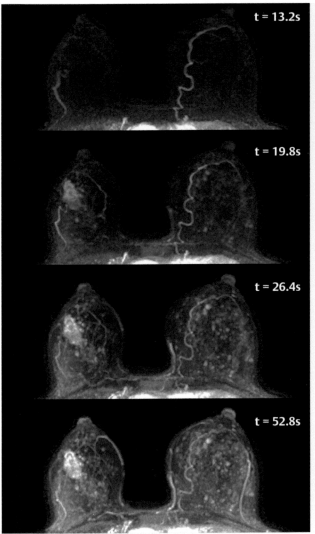

t = 13.2s

t = 19.8s

t = 26.4s

t = 52.8s

Fig. 6.2 Age 56 with a newly diagnosed invasive cancer in the right breast. Maximum intensity projections (MIPs) of ultra-fast subtraction images demonstrate an irregular mass in the central right breast with feeding vessels. Marked nodular parenchymal enhancement is noted in this case, with the cancer best seen on the 19.8 s image. The MIP images were generated from subtraction images obtained at 6.6 s temporal resolution, and the time following contract injection is labeled on each image.

must be 3 mm or less, the in-plane UF spatial resolution 2 to 3 mm, and the spatial resolution of the conventional contrast enhanced scan 0.8 mm. The in-plane resolution of the axial T2-weighted precontrast non–fat-suppressed sequence must be identical to the GRE sequence. An example of this type of acquisition is shown in ▶ Fig. 6.4. The technical specifics of this protocol at both field strengths are provided in ▶ Table 6.3 and ▶ Table 6.4.

Preliminary results using this protocol[62] demonstrate that enhancement in the breast during the first 20 to 40 seconds is very sparse; significant enhancement occurs in only about 5% of the volume of the breast. ▶ Fig. 6.3 demonstrates that only the primary invasive cancer and a few other small regions (shown in red) enhance during the first few seconds following arterial enhancement, suggesting that new approaches to further increase both temporal and spatial resolution without the need to use view sharing or compressed sensing methods could be used. For example, the field of view (FOV) can be set to a fraction of the FOV required to fully sample the object. Since early enhancement is sparse, it is unlikely that enhancing regions will overlap, and rare cases of overlap can be resolved by further analysis. Beginning at early times after injection and using an *aliasing factor* of

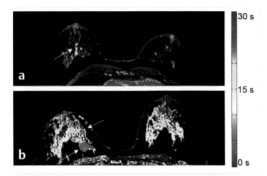

Fig. 6.3 Example of time-of-arrival (TOA) color maps. (a) Complex sclerosing lesion (radial scar), in the central right breast indicated by an arrow. (b) Invasive duct carcinoma, showing an index and satellite lesion (arrows) in a case with marked parenchymal enhancement. Color scale indicates the time-point at which voxels first arrive of the bolus. This image exemplifies the general trend observed, the malignant lesions had shorter TOA's on the average.

4, data can be acquired with an FOV that is one-fourth of the FOV needed to sample the entire object. As the enhancement becomes less sparse, at later times after injection (e.g., 20–60 seconds) the aliasing factor is slowly reduced until the object is fully sampled with an appropriate FOV (e.g., at 60 seconds after contrast media injection). This process is referred to as "*progressive aliasing*." With progressive aliasing, it is possible to perform complete sampling of enhancing regions at high temporal resolution combined with high spatial resolution, and in most cases without errors or loss of information as shown in ▶ Fig. 6.4a-f. This protocol can be combined with SENSE acceleration to further increase temporal and/or spatial resolution.

There is considerable work left to optimize methods for acquisition and analysis of UF DCE-MRI data, and to integrate UF imaging into AB-MRI protocols. However, the preliminary results

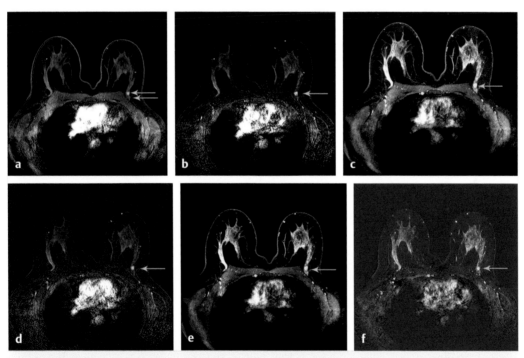

Fig. 6.4 AB-MR: Innovative protocol. A 42-year-old woman with a history of Paget disease of the left nipple, presented for magnetic resonance imaging evaluation. Axial T1-weighted fat suppressed ultrafast (UF) images were obtained in the first minute postcontrast injection followed by a standard 70-s acquisition. Selected axial images from the UF acquisition are shown (**a,b**), at 16 s and images at 24 s (**c,d**), postcontrast injection, respectively. Arrows indicate a 7-mm mass in the posterolateral aspect of the left breast (*arrows*); note minimal background parenchymal enhancement. Axial standard images (**e,f**) obtained at 140 s following the UF acquisition also demonstrate the small left breast mass (*arrows*). Subsequent histology yielded invasive ductal carcinoma grade 3.

Table 6.3 Ultrafast AB-MR screening protocol 1.5 T (Philips)

1. VISTA (non–fat-suppressed T2 weighted)

1. Precontrast masks, ultrafast DCE-MRI during the first minute postcontrast, followed by standard DCE-MRI for 1 min only

Parameters			
	VISTA	ultrafast DCE-MRI	DCE-MRI
Geometry	3D axial	3D axial	3D axial
FOV (mm)	320–400	320	320–400
Spatial resolution/ interpolated (mm)	0.8/0.8	1.5/0.8	0.8/0.7
Slice thickness/interpolated (mm)	2.0/1.0	3.5/1.75	2.0/1.0
Number of slices	200	100	175
Slice oversample	default	1	1.0
Slice gap (mm)	N/A	N/A	N/A
SENSE acceleration	3×2	4×2	2.5×2.0
TR (ms)	2000	4.7	5.5
TE (ms)	368	2.3	2.7
Flip angle (degrees)	90	12	12
Fast imaging mode	TSE	TFE	TFE
Fast imaging factor	120	21	44
Fat suppression	None	SPAIR	SPAIR
Partial Fourier imaging	no	0.70×0.85	No
k-space sampling	Cartesian	Cartesian	Cartesian
Number of averages	1	1	1
Duration (m:s)	2:32	2:03	5:24
Temporal resolution (m:s)	N/A	0:08.1	0:54
b values (s/mm²)	N/A	N/A	N/A

Abbreviations: AB-MR, abbreviated breast magnetic resonance imaging; DCE-MRI, dynamic contrast-enhanced MRI; FOV, field of view; SPAIR, Short scar periareola inferior pedicle reduction; TE, echo time; TFE, turbo field echo; TR, repetition time; TSE, turbo spin echo.
Notes: Parameters for VISTA and DCE-MRI are standard clinical parameters. No special consideration is needed beyond optimization for image quality in given time. Ultrafast DCE-MRI, voxel size, and SENSE factors are increased as much as possible with maintenance of good image quality.

from the UC group[59,61,62] and other laboratories[60] clearly demonstrate the potential of this method. Abbreviated MRI protocols that combine UF methods with conventional high-resolution postcontrast scans, as well as T2-weighted images, can provide radiologists with the outstanding morphologic detail they are accustomed to with a non–fat-saturated technique, combined with increased sensitivity to lesion morphology and physiology.

Table 6.4 Ultrafast AB-MR screening protocol 3.0 T (Philips)

1. VISTA (non–fat-suppressed T2 weighted)

1. Precontrast masks, ultrafast DCE-MRI during the first minute postcontrast, followed by standard DCE-MRI for 1 minute only (four more DCE-MRI acquisitions for a diagnostic study)

Parameters

	VISTA	Fast DCE-MRI	DCE-MRI
Geometry	3D axial	3D axial	3D axial
FOV (mm)	320–400	330	320–400
Spatial resolution/interpolated (mm)	0.8/0.65	1.5/0.76	0.8/0.6
Slice thickness/interpolated (mm)	1.6/0.8	3.0/1.5	1.6/0.8
Number of slices	250	115	250
Slice oversample	1.33	1	1.0
Slice gap (mm)	N/A	N/A	N/A
SENSE acceleration	3 × 2	4 × 2	2.5 × 2.0
TR (ms)	2000	3.1	4.8
TE (ms)	221	1.58	2.4
Flip angle (degrees)	90	10	10
Fast imaging mode	TSE	TFE	TFE
Fast imaging factor	120	25	27
Fat suppression	None	SPAIR	SPAIR
Partial Fourier imaging	No	0.75 × 0.85	0.85 × 1.0
k-space sampling	Cartesian	Cartesian	Cartesian
Number of averages	1	1	1
Duration (m:s)	3:44	1:35	5:13
Temporal resolution (m:s)	N/A	0:07.2	1:02
b values (s/mm²)	N/A	N/A	N/A

Abbreviations: AB-MR, abbreviated breast magnetic resonance imaging; DCE-MRI, dynamic contrast-enhanced MRI; FOV, field of view; SPAIR, short scar periareolar inferior pedicle reduction; TE, echo time; TFE, turbo field echo; TR, repetition time; TSE, turbo spin echo.
Notes: Parameters for VISTA and DCE-MRI are standard clinical parameters. No special consideration is needed beyond optimization for image quality in given time. Ultrafast DCE-MRI, voxel size, and SENSE factors are increased as much as possible with maintenance of good image quality.

6.8 Clinical Implementation of Abbreviated Breast Magnetic Resonance Imaging

6.8.1 Recruitment

The target population for screening with AB-MR will be those women at average to intermediate risk for breast cancer who have mammographically dense breasts. Women at intermediate risk are those with a 15 to < 20% lifetime risk of developing breast cancer. Several risk assessment models can be used to estimate lifetime breast cancer risk. All of these models depend heavily on family history, although consideration is also given to a variety of other risk factors such as age, reproductive history, and history of previous breast biopsy. An individual woman's risk estimate may vary with different models.

The Gail, Claus, and Tyrer–Cusick models are widely used and the *BRCA* Pro and BOADICEA models estimate the likelihood that a *BRCA* gene mutation is present.[69,70,71]

6.8.2 High-risk Women

The ACS has established recommendations,[21] based on the current research literature, recommending annual breast MRI as an adjunct to annual mammography for women over age 30 at high lifetime risk (> 20 to 25%) of developing breast cancer, based on risk-assessment computer models of key factors including family history. Annual breast MRI is also recommended for women who have a known *BRCA1* or *BRCA2* gene mutation,[71,72,73] have a first-degree relative with a *BRCA1* or *BRCA2* gene mutation and have not undergone genetic testing themselves, had radiation therapy to the chest when they were between the ages of 10 and 30 years,[74] or have certain syndromes (Li–Fraumeni, Cowden, or Bannayan–Riley–Ruvalcaba syndrome) either themselves or in a first-degree relative. Women who carry a mutation in these genes can have up to a 65% lifetime risk of developing breast cancer and also an increased risk of developing ovarian cancer.[21] Breast cancer risk for those receiving chest radiation at a young age has been shown to be highest for women treated during the time period from the1960s to mid-1970s, compared with those treated during the mid-late 1970s through the mid-1980s, when lower radiation doses were used.[74] The ACS and ACR guidelines recommend screening MRI as an adjunctive method for women with Hodgkin's disease or a history of mantle field radiation. Genetic counseling should be recommended for women who are found to be at increased risk of carrying a BRCA gene mutation. Women with a ≥ 20% lifetime risk for breast cancer should continue to undergo a standard full breast MRI and not an AB-MR until its role in this high-risk population has been fully established.

6.8.3 Women at Average and Moderate Risk (15 to < 20%) and Dense Breasts at Mammography

Isolated family history is not sufficient for inclusion into the high-risk category, because many women in the general population will have at least one relative with known breast cancer since about 12% of women will develop breast cancer at some

point in their lives. Breast cancer is common in the general population and it is important to recognize that only 5 to 10% of all breast cancers are thought to be hereditary.[20]

In recent years, 24 U.S. states have passed mandatory breast density notification legislation, and 6 more have introduced a bill.[74] These laws generally recommend consideration of adjunctive imaging screening methods for women with dense breast tissue at mammography. Physicians in clinical practice are now becoming aware that dense breast tissue is correlated with an increased risk of developing cancer and many are familiar with the legislative efforts aimed toward alerting their patients to the need for adjunctive screening studies. By Mammography Quality Standards Act (MQSA) national statute,[76] letters in lay language are sent to every woman screened by mammography, and these can include the density of tissue as reported by the radiologist. Such letters explain to the woman that she has dense breast tissue, that this is a common finding and is not abnormal, but that dense breast tissue can make it harder to find cancer on a mammogram and may increase her breast cancer risk. These lay reports raise awareness, suggest that women should discuss their own personal risk status with their referring doctor, and educate women to the advantages of adjunctive screening methods.[77] In order to inform women of the benefits of AB-MR, informational brochures could be placed in the mammography waiting room to introduce the concept of screening with MRI. As mentioned earlier, the sensitivity of breast MRI has been shown to be substantially higher than FFDM in women at moderate, mild, and average breast cancer risk and education and expansion of the use of AB-MR to this much larger population of women will be challenging. One approach might be to concentrate on the recruitment of women in an existing mammography screening practice, who have been shown by previous FFDM examination to have dense breast tissue. As previously noted, approximately 50% of the women will fall into this category (Breast Imaging Reporting and Data System [BI-RADS] categories C & D), where the sensitivity of mammography is diminished and overlapping dense tissue may increase the false-positive callback rate. Breast practice staff could review lists of scheduled screening mammograms in advance, and identify those women with a density classification of heterogeneously or extremely dense, as possible candidates for AB-MR adjunctive screening. Women with dense breast tissue could then be informed about the benefits of adjunctive MRI in addition to mammography screening, at the time of their routine mammography visit. The risks and benefits of MRI should be discussed, and printed literature distributed. In addition to the education of women undergoing mammography screening, education of the medical community regarding the utility of AB-MR will be needed. This educational effort should be a collaborative approach geared toward all physicians and allied health professionals involved in breast care. The further purpose would be to impart basic information, using publications, seminars, and educational conferences, to community hospitals and practices and local and national breast health organizations. It will be most important during the educational discussions to explain the distinction between a screening and a diagnostic MRI examination, emphasizing the benefits and efficiencies of AB-MR for breast cancer screening.

6.8.4 Equipment

The majority of breast DCE-MRI studies are still performed at magnetic field strengths of 1.5 T. However, recently there has been an increase in the use of higher field strength magnets (3.0 T), and dedicated breast coils with an increasing number of channels.[78]

A study by Elsamaloty et al reported increased sensitivity and specificity of DCE-MRI when performed at 3 T, finding values of 100 and 93.9%, respectively.[79] Another study by Rahbar et al showed that breast MRI at 3 T provided higher correlation with final pathology size of DCIS lesions compared to 1.5 T, and concluded that higher field strength may prove to be more accurate for assessment of disease extent in the preoperative setting.[80] These recent studies suggest that growing experience in scanning at higher field strength could lead to an overall increase of both sensitivity and specificity at MRI

6.8.5 Scheduling

Women scheduled for their first AB-MR appointment may wish for more information, have questions, and need to discuss the MRI study further before having their first screening MRI. These women could arrange for a discussion with either a qualified technologist or radiologist or her own referring physician, before the examination is scheduled. Details regarding payment methods should be arranged in advance of the appointment day.

Women may be scheduled for both their AB-MR and mammogram on the same visit. In order to streamline workflow for women undergoing both screening studies, coordination of scheduling to allow both imaging procedures on the same day could improve efficiency and lead to decreased costs and travel time. It should be possible to schedule an AB-MR appointment in a 20-minute time slot, allowing completion of both the MR and mammography examination within 1 hour. It is important to note that current ACS guidelines for breast MRI screening of high-risk women do not address the timing of MRI in conjunction with mammography. Therefore, referring physicians and radiologists need to develop screening protocols in their own community for women undergoing both AB-MR and mammography. These protocols could include women who schedule a mammogram every year in conjunction with AB-MR, and also women who prefer to alternate between AB-MR and mammography every 6 months.

Successful MRI is dependent on patient compliance and scheduling of postmenopausal women is achieved by routine methods because they are able to undergo DCE-MRI at any available time. Premenopausal women however should be scheduled according to their menstrual cycle, and should be scheduled preferentially on days 7 through 14 following the first day of the menstrual period if at all possible. When the background enhancement of the normal fibroglandular breast tissue is usually low, abnormal findings are more conspicuous, and false-positive findings are less frequent.[40,81,82,83] Scheduling of appointments for premenopausal women require flexibility, and appointments may need to be adjusted on an individual basis. If imaging is not performed during days 7 to 14 of the menstrual cycle, it is possible that lesions might be masked by the variable enhancement of fibroglandular tissue, thus reducing the accuracy of interpretation. Imaging in the fourth week of the cycle should be avoided whenever possible. Women using oral contraceptives should observe the menstrual cycle imaging recommendations. Certain women may experience irregular menses, particularly in the perimenopausal years, thus encountering difficulty in selecting the appropriate timing for their examination. In these instances, blood sampling for estimation of serum progesterone levels in order to determine the optimal time for breast MRI is helpful. This method may prove to be particularly useful when earlier examinations have been deemed nondiagnostic because of marked BPE.[84] It is interesting to note that a recent report indicates that hormone replacement therapy has negligible effect on the BPE of postmenopausal women who undergo MRI.[85]

6.8.6 Preparation

Adequate prior preparation is essential for efficient workflow on the day of imaging. Women should be prescreened, usually by telephone, for claustrophobia, allergic predisposition or history of prior reaction to contrast agents, presence of implantable devices, and history of renal disease. Attempts must be made to obtain all prior breast imaging examinations in advance,[86] and these studies should be uploaded onto the Picture Archiving and Communication System (PACS) before the patient arrives for her screening examinations.

6.8.7 Precautions and Contraindications

Some women experience mild claustrophobia when asked to enter and remain immobile inside the narrow chamber of the MRI device during the scanning period.[87] Claustrophobia is generally less severe when the woman is able to enter the scanner with her feet first rather than her head first, and moveable trolleys with built-in breast coils are especially useful in this regard. The majority of women are able to tolerate the study without difficulty, with the technologist providing verbal reassurance and encouraging the patient to remain immobile in between acquisition sequences, thus relieving anxiety during the procedure. Women who are extremely anxious may benefit from a discussion of the MRI procedure with a technologist or nurse and viewing of the scanning room and magnet before the examination. Women with severe claustrophobia may need sedation prior to the examination and this is usually arranged by consultation with her referring physician ahead of time.

Occasionally a referring physician may be concerned that a patient referred for MR examination may be too large to fit into the magnet bore and the breast coil. This issue can be resolved before scheduling the examination by inviting the woman to view the magnet and breast coil and attempting to position her in the device. If positioning and placement prove unsuccessful, then alternate screening methods should be employed.

All such questions and concerns should be managed if at all possible prior to the day of the screening appointment.

Allergic Predisposition

Women with a history of multiple allergies, bronchial asthma, or previous allergic reactions to gadolinium-based contrast media (GBCM) have a higher risk for allergic reactions and should discuss their allergic history with their referring physician. Precautionary methods can be taken in these cases including administration of antihistaminic and corticosteroid drugs prior to the examination. In women with serious allergic symptoms, a balance between the potential advantages of MRI and the potential risks of serious allergic reaction should be considered. It should be noted that there is no cross-reactivity between GBCM and iodinated contrast media.

Women with a history of moderate or severe allergic-like reactions to a specific GBCM may benefit from use of a different GBCM. It may also be prudent to premedicate for subsequent MR examinations, although there are no published studies to confirm that this approach is efficacious in reducing the likelihood of a repeat contrast reaction.

Foreign Bodies

Absolute contraindications to MRI include the presence of ferromagnetic intracranial aneurysm clips, and MR-incompatible implanted electronic devices such as pacemakers, implantable cardioverter defibrillators, and neurostimulators.

Women with intravascular stents or metal screws or plates for osteosynthesis can safely undergo breast MRI 6 weeks following surgical implantation. Women should be questioned as to whether they ever had an eye injury from a metal object (metal slivers, metal shavings, or other metal object). Orbital radiographs may be necessary to document the presence or absence of metal foreign bodies.

Women should inform the MRI technologists or nurses if they have any tattoos or permanent makeup, including tattooed eyeliner. If the tattoos are extensive or very dark, they may contain iron pigments and experience radiofrequency (RF) heating of the tattooed tissue causing local burns. Burning may occur if the tissue in question is located within the volume in which the body coil is being used for RF transmission. Cold compresses or ice packs placed over the tattooed areas during scanning and may alleviate the heat effect if they remain locally applied throughout the MRI examination. For further information, please review the ACR Guidance Document on MR Safe Practices.[88]

Renal Function

GBCMs are extremely well tolerated by the vast majority of patients who undergo DCE-MRI. Acute adverse reactions are rare and are encountered at a lower frequency than is reported following administration of iodinated contrast media. AB-MR screening should be avoided in women with severely impaired renal function because injection of GBCM may lead to a rare condition known as nephrogenic systemic fibrosis.[89] Renal function testing is recommended within 30 days of the scheduled examination for women over the age of 60 and this can be accomplished by obtaining a serum creatinine level and estimating the glomerular filtration rate. Testing should also be obtained for younger women with a history of bladder or kidney disease, diabetes mellitus or cardiovascular disease.[90,91]

DCE-MRI is generally contraindicated in pregnant women and AB-MRI should be avoided during pregnancy and lactation.[92]

6.9 Imaging Procedure

On the day of the AB-MR, clear instructions and a complete explanation of the MR procedure should be given to the woman by a radiology technologist or nurse. She will be asked to fill out a detailed questionnaire before entering the scanning room to confirm that she has no contraindication(s) to the MR examination or to the contrast injection. She will then be directed to the dressing area where she will change into a patient gown, having removed her brassiere, jewelry, and any clothing zippers or other metallic objects. In the preparation room of the MRI suite, a technologist or nurse will explain that she will receive an injection into her vein during scanning, and venous access should then be established with placement of an intravenous line. She should also be informed that she might experience a warm or tingling sensation in her arm, possibly extending throughout her body, both during and following the injection. Emphasis should be placed on the importance of remaining still during the scanning period, thus avoiding motion artifact and the need for repeat examination. The technologist will position the woman prone on the MRI table with her breasts symmetrically placed into the wells of the coil and with the nipples positioned at the most inferior aspect of the coil, with markers applied if requested by the radiologist. Folds or overlapping of breast tissue at the edges of the coil should be avoided and slight breast compression may be used to reduce motion artifacts. The woman should be informed that the scanning procedure is intermittently noisy, and she can be given ear plugs, or earphones with a choice of music if she wishes, aimed to minimize the noise during image acquisition. A method of verbal communication between the woman and the technologist or radiologist should be established before scanning takes place, and an alarm system should be provided to the woman so that she is aware that when she activates the alarm, the procedure will be stopped and she will immediately receive assistance.

Following image acquisition, the intravenous line is removed, the puncture site is compressed, and the woman will then sit on the table for a moment and then be able to exit from the magnet room. Once the woman has dressed in her own clothes, she may be asked to remain in the department for about 15 minutes to check for any possible delayed reaction to the GBCM before leaving the facility.

6.10 Reporting

The AB-MRI screening report should follow the BI-RADS developed by the ACR.[93] In addition to lesion characterization, the report must include the specific MR technique used, in summary form, and the type and amount of GBCM administered. The AB-MR report should include the volume of fibroglandular tissue, the amount of BPE, and when appropriate, the day or the week of the menstrual cycle on which the study was obtained.

Biopsy is usually indicated for new, isolated lesions diagnosed as BI-RADS 4 or 5. It is important to note that 50 to 70% of MRI findings requiring biopsy prove to be benign.[94] Before recommending an MR-guided biopsy, re-evaluation of prior mammograms and targeted mammographic or ultrasound views of the region of MR abnormality may allow biopsy of the MRI-detected lesion using mammographic or ultrasound guidance.

Although results are variable across different studies, about 60% of lesions initially detected at

MRI can be identified with MRI-directed or "second-look"-targeted ultrasound.[95,96] In these instances, percutaneous needle biopsy using ultrasound guidance can be performed, a faster and cheaper procedure than MR-guided biopsy. Caution is needed when searching with ultrasound for small MR-detected lesions such as small < 5 mm foci or masses, or small < 10 mm linear areas of nonmass enhancement. Confident correlative diagnosis of these small lesions at ultrasound may be challenging and MR-guided biopsy is often the preferable initial guidance method in these cases. If an MR-detected lesion is not identified at targeted ultrasound, then an MR-guided biopsy is indicated. For practices without the capability of MR-guided biopsy, the patient should be referred to a facility able to perform this procedure under a prearranged practice agreement. Careful correlation of pathology biopsy results with imaging findings is essential for accurate diagnosis.

Short-term follow-up, a BI-RADS 3 assessment, may be recommended instead of biopsy for a lesion perceived as having low malignancy probability and the expectation of no adverse therapeutic effect resulting from a short delay in cancer diagnosis. BI-RADS 3 lesions, a special diagnostic category carefully described initially at mammography with a likelihood of malignancy below 2%,[97] are not yet fully elucidated at MRI. Category 3 assessment requires repeat MRI examination within 6 months, again at 1 year and then if considered unchanged, resumption of yearly screening. MR-detected lesions may disappear, decrease, or remain unchanged in size without any new sign of malignancy, and these lesions can be downgraded to benign (BI-RADS 2) without the need for biopsy.

Caution should be given when applying a BI-RADS 3 lesion assessment to high-risk women in an MR screening program, because the malignancy risk in this cohort may be higher than 2%.[98,99] It is often helpful to initiate a discussion between the woman and her radiologist and/or referring physician, as to whether watchful waiting with a follow-up breast MRI within 6 months or a biopsy should be considered, and in some cases the woman will elect biopsy rather than follow-up.

6.10.1 Audit

The recommendations and results of subsequent biopsies based on results from AB-MR should be recorded to determine the cancer yield, PPV, recall rate, interval cancer rate, and frequency of recommendations for short-term follow-up. Although breast MRI has significant increased sensitivity and can detect smaller tumors than mammography, it has limitations. The overall sensitivity of breast MRI for breast cancer is approximately 90%. Missed cancers are usually either very small or do not exhibit sufficient contrast enhancement. Sensitivity for detection of duct carcinoma in situ (DCIS), a noninvasive lesion and a nonobligate precursor of invasive cancer, is variable, and lesions with a lower pathological grade (G1) can be missed at MRI.[17] Recall rates for additional imaging and for biopsy have been noted to be higher with MRI in high-risk populations, ranging from 8 to 17% for imaging and 3 to 15% for biopsy.[18,19,100,101,102] Recall rates have been shown to decrease with subsequent rounds of screening and factors contributing to the sensitivity and recall rates include the technical quality of the acquisition and the experience of the reader. An audit should be conducted as part of routine MRI screening practice.

6.11 Costs

Although MRI may eventually become the routine method used in breast cancer surveillance, the high cost of the examination is currently a major factor in the restriction of its use, and studies of the cost-effectiveness of adding breast MRI to annual mammography have only incorporated those women deemed to be at the highest risk of developing breast cancer.

Plevritis et al reported that the addition of breast MRI was cost-effective in both *BRCA1* and *BRCA2* mutation carriers.[102] They also showed that although the cost benefits were greatest in patients aged 40 to 49 years for both mutation types, the cost per quality-adjusted life year (QALY) was greater in women with *BRCA1* mutations and varied greatly with age. The *BRCA1* group was found to have a higher risk for cancer, including more aggressive cancers, compared with *BRCA2* mutations, resulting in an increased cost savings. Ahern et al studied various options for integrating mammography and MRI schedules into a screening protocol for women with a strong family history of breast cancer and a lifetime risk of > 25% or higher. Using current costs of MRI examinations and an incremental cost-effectiveness ratio of $100,000 per QALY, they found that the most cost-effective strategy was an alternating schedule of MRI and mammography examinations, plus a clinical breast exam, every year from age 30 to 74. For those women with a 50% lifetime risk, the recommended strategy was to follow the same screening protocol but to alternate these examinations every 6 months, provided there was a 70% reduction in MRI costs. At 75% risk, the recommended strategy became biennial MRI combined with mammography plus clinical breast exam every 6 months.[103,104] When considering costs, additional investigations need to be taken into account, such as repeat MRI examinations, targeted ultrasound studies, and percutaneous biopsies of screen-detected breast lesions. These additional costs are greater for women at lower breast cancer risk; therefore, the cost-effectiveness of MRI screening has been questioned for women who are not at increased risk. It is apparent that in order to screen women at intermediate or average risk, the cost of the MRI examination needs to be lower, the examination shorter, and the workflow seamless. Health care reimbursement for breast MRI screening is variable among differing developed countries across the world, and additional economic studies comparing the downstream costs of AB-MR breast screening with WBUS are needed.

6.12 Summary

Screening for breast cancer has long been a topic of debate and a source of high anxiety for women. Implementation of AB-MR technique as an adjunctive method to screening mammography is an innovative and challenging endeavor. If this method proves to be successful and results in the detection of significantly more high-grade cancers in the MR screened group than mammography, while also reducing interval cancers, then women will be able to choose individualized breast cancer screening regimens devised according to their risk estimates and breast density. Implementation of AB-MR into routine screening practice will present a challenging task for all physicians and allied professionals involved in breast cancer care, but the rewards should benefit women by decreasing mortality from breast cancer.

References

[1] American Cancer Society. Breast cancer prevention and early detection. http://www.cancer.org/acs/groups/cid/documents/webcontent/003165-pdf.pdf. Accessed June 20, 2015

[2] Tabár L, Vitak B, Chen TH, et al. Swedish two-county trial: impact of mammographic screening on breast cancer mortality during 3 decades. Radiology. 2011; 260(3):658–663

[3] Tabár L, Fagerberg CJ, Gad A, et al. Reduction in mortality from breast cancer after mass screening with mammography. Randomised trial from the Breast Cancer Screening Working Group of the Swedish National Board of Health and Welfare. Lancet. 1985; 1(8433):829–832

[4] Institute of Medicine. Saving Women's Lives: Integration and Innovation: A Framework for progress in Early Detection and diagnosis of Breast Cancer. Washington, DC: National Academies Press; 2005

[5] Ciatto S, Houssami N, Bernardi D, et al. Integration of 3D digital mammography with tomosynthesis for population breast-cancer screening (STORM): a prospective comparison study. Lancet Oncol. 2013; 14(7):583–589

[6] Skaane P, Bandos AI, Gullien R, et al. Prospective trial comparing full-field digital mammography (FFDM) versus combined FFDM and tomosynthesis in a population-based screening programme using independent double reading with arbitration. Eur Radiol. 2013; 23(8):2061–2071

[7] Skaane P, Bandos AI, Gullien R, et al. Comparison of digital mammography alone and digital mammography plus tomosynthesis in a population-based screening program. Radiology. 2013; 267(1):47–56

[8] Friedewald SM, Rafferty EA, Rose SL, et al. Breast cancer screening using tomosynthesis in combination with digital mammography. JAMA. 2014; 311(24):2499–2507

[9] Fletcher SW, Elmore JG. Clinical practice. Mammographic screening for breast cancer. N Engl J Med. 2003; 348 (17):1672–1680

[10] Institute for Health Quality and Ethics Analysis. 10,000 deaths a year due to false and misleading mammogram reports. http://instituteforhealthqualityandethics.com/uploads/120120_Deaths_Due_to_False_Mammogram_Results.pdf. Accessed June 15, 2015

[11] Price ER, Hargreaves J, Lipson JA, et al. The California breast density information group: a collaborative response to the issues of breast density, breast cancer risk, and breast density notification legislation. Radiology. 2013; 269(3):887–892

[12] Berg WA, Blume JD, Cormack JB, et al. ACRIN 6666 Investigators. Combined screening with ultrasound and mammography vs mammography alone in women at elevated risk of breast cancer. JAMA. 2008; 299(18):2151–2163

[13] Berg WA, Zhang Z, Lehrer D, et al. ACRIN 6666 Investigators. Detection of breast cancer with addition of annual screening ultrasound or a single screening MRI to mammography in women with elevated breast cancer risk. JAMA. 2012; 307 (13):1394–1404

[14] Boetes C, Barentsz JO, Mus RD, et al. MR characterization of suspicious breast lesions with a gadolinium-enhanced TurboFLASH subtraction technique. Radiology. 1994; 193 (3):777–781

[15] Orel SG, Schnall MD. MR imaging of the breast for the detection, diagnosis, and staging of breast cancer. Radiology. 2001; 220(1):13–30

[16] Liu PF, Debatin JF, Caduff RF, Kacl G, Garzoli E, Krestin GP. Improved diagnostic accuracy in dynamic contrast enhanced MRI of the breast by combined quantitative and qualitative analysis. Br J Radiol. 1998; 71(845):501–509

[17] Kriege M, Brekelmans CT, Boetes C, et al. Magnetic Resonance Imaging Screening Study Group. Efficacy of MRI and mammography for breast-cancer screening in women with a familial or genetic predisposition. N Engl J Med. 2004; 351 (5):427–437

[18] Kuhl CK, Schrading S, Leutner CC, et al. Mammography, breast ultrasound, and magnetic resonance imaging for surveillance of women at high familial risk for breast cancer. J Clin Oncol. 2005; 23(33):8469–8476

[19] Leach MO, Boggis CR, Dixon AK, et al. MARIBS study group. Screening with magnetic resonance imaging and mammography of a UK population at high familial risk of breast cancer: a prospective multicentre cohort study (MARIBS). Lancet. 2005; 365(9473):1769–1778

[20] American Cancer Society. Breast cancer prevention and early detection. http://www.cancer.org/acs/groups/cid/documents/webcontent/003165-pdf. Accessed July 1, 2015

[21] Saslow D, Boetes C, Burke W, et al. American Cancer Society Breast Cancer Advisory Group. American Cancer Society guidelines for breast screening with MRI as an adjunct to mammography. CA Cancer J Clin. 2007; 57(2):75–89

[22] American College of Radiology. ACR practice parameter for the performance of contrast-enhanced magnetic resonance imaging (MRI) of the breast. http://www.acr.org/~/media/2a0eb28eb59041e2825179afb72ef624.pdf. Accessed July 1, 2015

[23] Brennan S, Liberman L, Dershaw DD, Morris E. Breast MRI screening of women with a personal history of breast cancer. AJR Am J Roentgenol. 2010; 195(2):510–516

[24] McCormack VA, dos Santos Silva I. Breast density and parenchymal patterns as markers of breast cancer risk: a meta-analysis. Cancer Epidemiol Biomarkers Prev. 2006; 15(6):1159–1169

[25] Simpson JF. Update on atypical epithelial hyperplasia and ductal carcinoma in situ. Pathology. 2009; 41(1):36–39

[26] Hartmann LC, Degnim AC, Santen RJ, Dupont WD, Ghosh K. Atypical hyperplasia of the breast–risk assessment and management options. N Engl J Med. 2015; 372(1):78–89

[27] Hartmann LC, Radisky DC, Frost MH, et al. Understanding the premalignant potential of atypical hyperplasia through its natural history: a longitudinal cohort study. Cancer Prev Res (Phila). 2014; 7(2):211–217

[28] Page DL, Schuyler PA, Dupont WD, Jensen RA, Plummer WD, Jr, Simpson JF. Atypical lobular hyperplasia as a unilateral predictor of breast cancer risk: a retrospective cohort study. Lancet. 2003; 361(9352):125–129

[29] Sung JS, Malak SF, Bajaj P, Alis R, Dershaw DD, Morris EA. Screening breast MR imaging in women with a history of lobular carcinoma in situ. Radiology. 2011; 261(2):414–420

[30] Londero V, Zuiani C, Linda A, Girometti R, Bazzocchi M, Sardanelli F. High-risk breast lesions at imaging-guided needle biopsy: usefulness of MRI for treatment decision. AJR Am J Roentgenol. 2012; 199(2):W240–50

[31] Schrading S, Kuhl CK. MRI screening of women at average risk of breast cancer. J Clin Oncol. 2013; 31 Suppl 26:21

[32] Mango VL, Morris EA, David Dershaw D, et al. Abbreviated protocol for breast MRI: are multiple sequences needed for cancer detection? Eur J Radiol. 2015; 84(1):65–70

[33] Kuhl CK, Schrading S, Strobel K, Schild HH, Hilgers RD, Bieling HB. Abbreviated breast magnetic resonance imaging (MRI): first postcontrast subtracted images and maximum-intensity projection-a novel approach to breast cancer screening with MRI. J Clin Oncol. 2014; 32(22):2304–2310

[34] Bird RE, McLelland R. How to initiate and operate a low-cost screening mammography center. Radiology. 1986; 161(1):43–47

[35] MRI Accreditation - American College of Radiology. www.acr.org/Quality-Safety/Accreditation/MRI. Accessed July 1 2015

[36] Kuhl CK, Mielcareck P, Klaschik S, et al. Dynamic breast MR imaging: are signal intensity time course data useful for differential diagnosis of enhancing lesions? Radiology. 1999; 211(1):101–110

[37] Buadu LD, Murakami J, Murayama S, et al. Breast lesions: correlation of contrast medium enhancement patterns on MR images with histopathologic findings and tumor angiogenesis. Radiology. 1996; 200(3):639–649

[38] Delille JP, Slanetz PJ, Yeh ED, Kopans DB, Garrido L. Physiologic changes in breast magnetic resonance imaging during the menstrual cycle: perfusion imaging, signal enhancement, and influence of the T1 relaxation time of breast tissue. Breast J. 2005; 11(4):236–241

[39] Amarosa AR, McKellop J, Klautau Leite AP, et al. Evaluation of the kinetic properties of background parenchymal enhancement throughout the phases of the menstrual cycle. Radiology. 2013; 268(2):356–365

[40] DeMartini WB, Liu F, Peacock S, Eby PR, Gutierrez RL, Lehman CD. Background parenchymal enhancement on breast MRI: impact on diagnostic performance. AJR Am J Roentgenol. 2012; 198(4):W373–W380

[41] Kuhl C. The current status of breast MR imaging. Part I. Choice of technique, image interpretation, diagnostic accuracy, and transfer to clinical practice. Radiology. 2007; 244(2):356–378

[42] Jansen SA, Shimauchi A, Zak L, et al. Kinetic curves of malignant lesions are not consistent across MRI systems: need for improved standardization of breast dynamic contrast-enhanced MRI acquisition. AJR Am J Roentgenol. 2009; 193(3):832–839

[43] Pineda FD, Medved M, Fan X, et al. Comparison of dynamic contrast-enhanced MRI parameters of breast lesions at 1.5 and 3.0T: a pilot study. Br J Radiol. 2015; 88(1049):20150021

[44] Tofts PS. Modeling tracer kinetics in dynamic Gd-DTPA MR imaging. J Magn Reson Imaging. 1997; 7(1):91–101

[45] Tofts PS, Brix G, Buckley DL, et al. Estimating kinetic parameters from dynamic contrast-enhanced T(1)-weighted MRI of a diffusable tracer: standardized quantities and symbols. J Magn Reson Imaging. 1999; 10(3):223–232

[46] Medved M, Karczmar G, Yang C, et al. Semiquantitative analysis of dynamic contrast enhanced MRI in cancer patients: Variability and changes in tumor tissue over time. J Magn Reson Imaging. 2004; 20(1):122–128

[47] Evelhoch JL, LoRusso PM, He Z, et al. Magnetic resonance imaging measurements of the response of murine and human tumors to the vascular-targeting agent ZD6126. Clin Cancer Res. 2004; 10(11):3650–3657

[48] Fan X, Haney CR, Mustafi D, et al. Use of a reference tissue and blood vessel to measure the arterial input function in DCEMRI. Magn Reson Med. 2010; 64(6):1821–1826

[49] Heisen M, Fan X, Buurman J, van Riel NA, Karczmar GS, ter Haar Romeny BM. The use of a reference tissue arterial input function with low-temporal-resolution DCE-MRI data. Phys Med Biol. 2010; 55(16):4871–4883

[50] Yang C, Karczmar GS, Medved M, Stadler WM. Estimating the arterial input function using two reference tissues in dynamic contrast-enhanced MRI studies: fundamental concepts and simulations. Magn Reson Med. 2004; 52(5):1110–1117

[51] Yang C, Karczmar GS, Medved M, Stadler WM. Multiple reference tissue method for contrast agent arterial input function estimation. Magn Reson Med. 2007; 58(6):1266–1275

[52] Pineda FD, Medved M, Fan X, Karczmar GS. B1 and T1 mapping of the breast with a reference tissue method. Magn Reson Med. 2016; 75(4):1565–1573

[53] Sung K, Daniel BL, Hargreaves BA. Transmit B1+field inhomogeneity and T1 estimation errors in breast DCE-MRI at 3 tesla. J Magn Reson Imaging. 2013; 38(2):454–459

[54] Sung K, Saranathan M, Daniel BL, Hargreaves BA. Simultaneous T(1) and B(1) (+) mapping using reference region variable flip angle imaging. Magn Reson Med. 2013; 70(4):954–961

[55] Rohrer M, Bauer H, Mintorovitch J, Requardt M, Weinmann HJ. Comparison of magnetic properties of MRI contrast media solutions at different magnetic field strengths. Invest Radiol. 2005; 40(11):715–724

[56] Walker-Samuel S, Leach MO, Collins DJ. Evaluation of response to treatment using DCE-MRI: the relationship between initial area under the gadolinium curve (IAUGC) and quantitative pharmacokinetic analysis. Phys Med Biol. 2006; 51(14):3593–3602

[57] Leach MO, Brindle KM, Evelhoch JL, et al. Pharmacodynamic/Pharmacokinetic Technologies Advisory Committee, Drug Development Office, Cancer Research UK. The assessment of antiangiogenic and antivascular therapies in early-stage clinical trials using magnetic resonance imaging: issues and recommendations. Br J Cancer. 2005; 92 (9):1599–1610

[58] Kuhl CK, Schrading S, Strobel K, Schild HH, Hilgers RD, Bieling HB. Abbreviated breast magnetic resonance imaging (MRI): first postcontrast subtracted images and maximum-intensity projection-a novel approach to breast cancer screening with MRI. J Clin Oncol. 2014; 32(22):2304–2310

[59] Jansen SA, Fan X, Medved M, et al. Characterizing early contrast uptake of ductal carcinoma in situ with high temporal resolution dynamic contrast-enhanced MRI of the breast: a pilot study. Phys Med Biol. 2010; 55(19):N473–N485

[60] Pinker K, Grabner G, Bogner W, et al. A combined high temporal and high spatial resolution 3 Tesla MR imaging protocol for the assessment of breast lesions: initial results. Invest Radiol. 2009; 44(9):553–558

[61] Pineda FD. Semi-Quantitative and Quantitative Dynamic Contrast-Enhanced MRI of the Breast, in Medical Physics. Chicago, IL: University of Chicago;2015

[62] Pineda F, Tsuchiya K, Abe H, et al. Characterization of Breast Lesion Kinetics with Accelerated DCE-MRI Using Conventional Sampling Methods. Chicago, IL: Radiological Society of North America;2015

[63] Ramsay E, Causer P, Hill K, Plewes D. Adaptive bilateral breast MRI using projection reconstruction time-resolved imaging of contrast kinetics. J Magn Reson Imaging. 2006; 24(3):617–624

[64] Tudorica LA, Oh KY, Roy N, et al. A feasible high spatiotemporal resolution breast DCE-MRI protocol for clinical settings. Magn Reson Imaging. 2012; 30(9):1257–1267

[65] Kershaw LE, Cheng HL. A general dual-bolus approach for quantitative DCE-MRI. Magn Reson Imaging. 2011; 29 (2):160–166

[66] Chan RW, Ramsay EA, Cheung EY, Plewes DB. The influence of radial undersampling schemes on compressed sensing reconstruction in breast MRI. Magn Reson Med. 2012; 67 (2):363–377

[67] Smith DS, Welch EB, Li X, et al. Quantitative effects of using compressed sensing in dynamic contrast enhanced MRI. Phys Med Biol. 2011; 56(15):4933–4946

[68] http://www.cancer.org/cancer/breastcancer/moreinformation/breastcancerearlydetection/breast-cancer-early-detection-acs-recs. Accessed July 1, 2015

[69] http://www.cancer.gov/types/breast/hp/breast-ovarian-genetics-pdq#section/_1. Accessed July 1, 2015

[70] Campeau PM, Foulkes WD, Tischkowitz MD. Hereditary breast cancer: new genetic developments, new therapeutic avenues. Hum Genet. 2008; 124(1):31–42

[71] Chen S, Parmigiani G. Meta-analysis of BRCA1 and BRCA2 penetrance. J Clin Oncol. 2007; 25(11):1329–1333

[72] Wahner-Roedler DL, Nelson DF, Croghan IT, et al. Risk of breast cancer and breast cancer characteristics in women treated with supradiaphragmatic radiation for Hodgkin lymphoma: Mayo Clinic experience. Mayo Clin Proc. 2003; 78 (6):708–715

[73] Tinger A, Wasserman TH, Klein EE, et al. The incidence of breast cancer following mantle field radiation therapy as a function of dose and technique. Int J Radiat Oncol Biol Phys. 1997; 37(4):865–870

[74] Slanetz PJ, Freer PE, Birdwell RL. Breast-density legislation-practical considerations. N Engl J Med. 2015; 372(7):593–595

[75] The Mammography Quality Standards Act Final Regulations: Modifications and Additions to Policy Guidance Help System #9. www.fda.gov/.../MammographyQualitySt. Accessed September 1, 2015

[76] www.fda.gov/downloads/MedicalDevices/.../ucm094441. pdf. Accessed July 1, 2015

[77] http://www.acr.org/Quality-Safety/Accreditation/Mammography/Lay-Letters. Accessed July 1, 2015

[78] Bassett LW, Dhaliwal SG, Eradat J, et al. National trends and practices in breast MRI. AJR Am J Roentgenol. 2008; 191 (2):332–339

[79] Elsamaloty H, Elzawawi MS, Mohammad S, Herial N. Increasing accuracy of detection of breast cancer with 3-T MRI. AJR Am J Roentgenol. 2009; 192(4):1142–1148

[80] Rahbar H, DeMartini WB, Lee AY, Partridge SC, Peacock S, Lehman CD. Accuracy of 3 T versus 1.5 T breast MRI for preoperative assessment of extent of disease in newly diagnosed DCIS. Eur J Radiol. 2015; 84(4):611–616

[81] Kuhl CK, Bieling HB, Gieseke J, et al. Healthy premenopausal breast parenchyma in dynamic contrast-enhanced MR imaging of the breast: normal contrast medium enhancement and cyclical-phase dependency. Radiology. 1997; 203 (1):137–144

[82] Kajihara M, Goto M, Hirayama Y, et al. Effect of the menstrual cycle on background parenchymal enhancement in breast MR imaging. Magn Reson Med Sci. 2013; 12(1):39–45

[83] Ellis RL. Optimal timing of breast MRI examinations for premenopausal women who do not have a normal menstrual cycle. AJR Am J Roentgenol. 2009; 193(6):1738–1740

[84] Hegenscheid K, Schmidt CO, Seipel R, et al. Contrast enhancement kinetics of normal breast parenchyma in dynamic MR mammography: effects of menopausal status, oral contraceptives, and postmenopausal hormone therapy. Eur Radiol. 2012; 22(12):2633–2640

[85] Morris EA, Comstock CE, Lee CH, et al. ACR BI-RADS magnetic resonance imaging. In: D'Orsi CJ, Ed. ACR BI-RADS Atlas: Breast Imaging Reporting and Data System. 5th ed. Reston, VA: American College of Radiology; 2013

[86] Eshed I, Althoff CE, Hamm B, Hermann KG. Claustrophobia and premature termination of magnetic resonance imaging examinations. J Magn Reson Imaging. 2007; 26(2):401–404

[87] Kanal E, Barkovich AJ, Bell C, et al. Expert Panel on MR Safety. ACR guidance document on MR safe practices: 2013. J Magn Reson Imaging. 2013; 37(3):501–530

[88] Thomsen HS, Morcos SK, Almén T, et al. ESUR Contrast Medium Safety Committee. Nephrogenic systemic fibrosis and gadolinium-based contrast media: updated ESUR Contrast Medium Safety Committee guidelines. Eur Radiol. 2013; 23 (2):307–318

[89] ACR Committee on Drugs and Contrast Media. ACR Manual on Contrast Media Version 10.1. Reston, VA: American College of Radiology; 2015

[90] US Food and Drug Administration. Questions and answers on gadolinium-based contrast agents. Updated July 30, 2014. http://www.fda.gov/Drugs/DrugSafety/DrugSafety-Newsletter/ucm142889.htm. Accessed July 16, 2015

[91] Cova MA, Stacul F, Quaranta R, et al. Radiological contrast media in the breastfeeding woman: a position paper of the Italian Society of Radiology (SIRM), the Italian Society of Paediatrics (SIP), the Italian Society of Neonatology (SIN) and the Task Force on Breastfeeding, Ministry of Health, Italy. Eur Radiol. 2014; 24(8):2012–2022

[92] American College of Radiology (ACR) Breast Imaging Reporting and Data System Atlas. (BI-RADS Atlas). Reston, VA: American College of Radiology; 2013. http://www.acr.org/

[93] Smith H, Chetlen AL, Schetter S, Mack J, Watts M, Zhu JJ. PPV (3) of suspicious breast MRI findings. Acad Radiol. 2014; 21 (12):1553–1562

[94] Abe H, Schmidt RA, Shah RN, et al. MR-directed ("Second-Look") ultrasound examination for breast lesions detected initially on MRI: MR and sonographic findings. AJR Am J Roentgenol. 2010; 194(2):370–377

[95] Spick C, Baltzer PA. Diagnostic utility of second-look US for breast lesions identified at MR imaging: systematic review and meta-analysis. Radiology. 2014; 273(2):401–409

[96] Sickles EA. Management of probably benign lesions of the breast. Radiology. 1994; 193(2):582–583

[97] Comstock C, Sung JS. BI-RADS 3 for magnetic resonance imaging. Magn Reson Imaging Clin N Am. 2013; 21 (3):561–570

[98] Spick C, Szolar DH, Baltzer PA, et al. Rate of malignancy in MRI-detected probably benign (BI-RADS 3) lesions. AJR Am J Roentgenol. 2014; 202(3):684–689

[99] Kuhl CK, Schrading S, Bieling HB, et al. MRI for diagnosis of pure ductal carcinoma in situ: a prospective observational study. Lancet. 2007; 370(9586):485–492

[100] Lehman CD, Blume JD, Weatherall P, et al. International Breast MRI Consortium Working Group. Screening women at high risk for breast cancer with mammography and magnetic resonance imaging. Cancer. 2005; 103(9):1898–1905

[101] Warner E, Plewes DB, Hill KA, et al. Surveillance of BRCA1 and BRCA2 mutation carriers with magnetic resonance imaging, ultrasound, mammography, and clinical breast examination. JAMA. 2004; 292(11):1317–1325

[102] Plevritis SK, Kurian AW, Sigal BM, et al. Cost-effectiveness of screening BRCA1/2 mutation carriers with breast magnetic resonance imaging. JAMA. 2006; 295(20):2374–2384

[103] Ahern CH, Shih YC, Dong W, Parmigiani G, Shen Y. Cost-effectiveness of alternative strategies for integrating MRI into breast cancer screening for women at high risk. Br J Cancer. 2014; 111(8):1542–1551

[104] Taneja C, Edelsberg J, Weycker D, Guo A, Oster G, Weinreb J. Cost effectiveness of breast cancer screening with contrast-enhanced MRI in high-risk women. J Am Coll Radiol. 2009; 6(3):171–179

7 Interpretation Guidelines

Janice S. Sung and Constance D. Lehman

7.1 Introduction

The concept of an abbreviated breast Magnetic Resonance Imaging (AB-MR) is to reduce the time and cost of a screening breast MRI in order to allow more women to have access to MRI while maintaining high sensitivity for breast cancer detection and high specificity. Although somewhat arbitrary and dependent on the local reimbursement rates, a scan time of 10 minutes or less compared with a 20- to 40-minute non-abbreviated full breast MRI would reduce the cost of AB-MR so that it is comparable to the cost of combined screening with mammography and whole breast ultrasound.

For cancer detection, the minimum sequences of an AB-MR protocol must include a localization scan and one pre- and one postcontrast T1-weighted acquisition. The in-plane resolution should be 1 mm or less, and the slice thickness should be less than 3 mm. Derived maximum intensity projection (MIP) and subtraction MIP images may be utilized to facilitate interpretation. Although not required, a T2-weighted sequence is highly encouraged in order to reduce false positives. Additional sequences, such as ultrafast perfusion imaging or a second postcontrast series, may also be included as long as the acquisition time is maintained at 10 minutes or less. The interpretation guidelines presented in this chapter are based on an AB-MR protocol that includes a pre- and postcontrast fat-saturated T1-weighted image and a fat-saturated T2-weighted sequence.

Lesion enhancement is due to the diffusion and accumulation of gadolinium in the interstitial spaces of lesions and within ducts. Tumor angiogenesis plays a fundamental role in local tumor growth, invasion, and progression to metastases.[1,2] As tumors outgrow their native blood supply, hypoxia ensues, which induces expression of multiple angiogenic factors such as vascular endothelial growth factor (VEGF). These factors induce the growth of existing capillaries and the formation of abnormal vessels that are leakier than native vessels. Increased enhancement of tumors relative to the normal surrounding parenchyma may result from both an increased supply through this proliferative network of vessels and their increased permeability. This increased early enhancement of tumors can be seen on both the AB-MR and a nonabbreviated MRI. Although initial early enhancement is characterized as slow, medium, or fast, there are no set criteria defining the actual threshold percentage increase in enhancement to classify early enhancement as slow, medium, or fast. However, invasive cancers usually demonstrate at least > 50% early enhancement.

Increased permeability of vessels associated with tumor angiogenesis also results in early washout of contrast from malignant lesions compared to the normal breast parenchyma. The delayed phase of enhancement refers to the pattern of enhancement following the first postcontrast series, and is described as persistent (or progressive), plateau, or washout. Lesions on MRI that demonstrate both a rapid initial uptake and delayed washout enhancement pattern raise suspicion for associated angiogenesis. In an abbreviated MRI protocol that utilizes only one single postcontrast scan, delayed enhancement kinetics, especially the presence of washout kinetics, cannot be evaluated and are not incorporated into AB-MR interpretation. In practice, the absence of delayed kinetic information should only have a minimal impact on sensitivity and specificity as MR interpretation is based predominantly on lesion morphology. Traditionally, the delayed kinetic pattern has been incorporated into lesion analysis after first evaluating morphology and composition (fat or fluid content on T1- and T2-weighted sequences).[3] In women with a comparison MRI, kinetics play an even smaller role, as any new unique lesion (i.e., new enhancing mass) will require biopsy regardless of the kinetic pattern.

The interpretation approach should also be tailored to the population being imaged. Patients that are at high risk (≥ 20–25% lifetime risk) are still recommended to have a breast MRI using a standard full protocol. Breast MRI performed with an abbreviated protocol is geared toward women with dense breasts that are at average to intermediate risk for breast cancer. The threshold for recommending biopsy or a follow-up should be higher with an AB-MR than when interpreting MRIs for high-risk screening as the likelihood of malignancy is less.

7.2 Approach to Interpretation

7.2.1 Assessment of Image Quality

Similar to mammography, the first step in AB-MR image interpretation is to assess image quality (Algorithm 1: Approach to MR Interpretation Readout[1]). This includes evaluating for adequate positioning, contrast administration, optimal technique, and motion artifact.

Proper positioning is essential in performing high-quality breast MRI. The MRI technologists should be trained in proper positioning. The patient should be positioned prone and the breast centered in a dedicated breast coil with the nipple in profile. Attention should be paid to include as much of the medial and axillary breast tissue as possible. Efforts should be made to ensure the patient is as comfortable as possible, which will reduce patient motion during the scan.

All breast MRI is based on the administration of intravenous gadolinium contrast in order to show increased relative enhancement of breast cancers relative to the normal parenchyma. Therefore, images should be assessed to confirm successful contrast administration. Contrast should be visible in the heart, blood vessels, and lymph nodes on the postcontrast images.

Fat saturation is highly recommended with the AB-MR protocol. Fat saturation should be uniform to avoid errors in interpretation. On fat-saturated T1-weighted images, the fat should appear gray and glandular tissue should maintain T1 signal. Glandular tissue that appears uniformly dark on the precontrast images suggests water suppression, which occurs if the suppression pulse is inadvertently applied to the water frequency peak and not the fat frequency peak.

Finally, postcontrast images and the subtraction series should be assessed for motion artifact. Many radiologists rely on the subtracted images (postcontrast series minus precontrast series), which display only areas of enhancement in the breast. The subtraction series are less distracting than the postcontrast series

where high signal areas may be due to either true enhancement or inherent high T1 signal such as proteinaceous debris or hemorrhage (▶ Fig. 7.1). However, the quality of subtracted images is significantly affected by patient motion, causing the unenhanced and contrast-enhanced images to be misaligned, leading to misregistration on the subtraction images. Patient motion may result in areas of pseudoenhancement on subtraction images. Findings on the subtraction images suggesting motion artifact include pseudoenhancement of the skin, areas of signal dropout, or an overall hazy appearance of the glandular tissue. Most MRI computer-aided detection (CAD) systems perform some form of image registration correction to improve alignment of sequences affected by slight patient motion and reduce subtraction artifact. Registration correction is particularly important for breast MRI studies in which fat suppression is not performed and subtraction images are heavily relied upon. Significant patient motion cannot be overcome by MRI CAD registration correction algorithms and may lead to erroneous assessments if interpretation is based on the subtraction images. In cases with significant patient motion, interpretation should be based on the source images rather than the subtracted images.

7.3 Global Assessment of Fibroglandular Tissue and Background Parenchymal Enhancement

The fifth edition of the Breast Imaging Reporting and Data System (BI-RADS) Atlas requires that each MR report contain a description of the amount of fibroglandular tissue present, as well as the level of the background parenchymal enhancement (BPE).[4]

The amount of fibroglandular tissues (FGT) refers to the amount of nonfatty, noncystic normal breast parenchyma. FGT may best be assessed on a non–fat-saturated T1-weighted image if one is performed. Otherwise, the fat-saturated T1-weighted images may be used. Similar to mammography, the amount of FGT is classified within one of four categories: almost entirely fat, scattered fibroglandular tissue, heterogeneous fibroglandular tissue, and extreme fibroglandular tissue based on the relative proportion of fat and glandular tissue.

---

[1] The Society of Breast MRI Interpretation Guidelines suggest a standardized method for abbreviated breast MRI interpretation. These algorithms are not meant to dictate individual case management decisions. The ultimate decision regarding AB-MR interpretation must be made by the interpreting radiologist in light of all the circumstances presented in an individual examination.

AB-MR Interpretation Overview

• Goal of AB-MR interpretation is to maintain high sensitivity and specificity
• In order to minimize false positives and short term follow ups, it is fundamental to identify only findings that are truly unique to the background parenchymal enhancement (BPE)
• Biopsy and short-term follow up should be reserved for lesions ≥3 mm in size

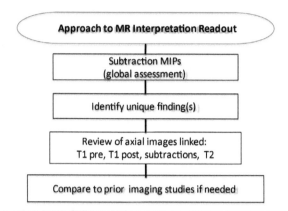

Algorithm 1 Approach to magnetic resonance interpretation readout. (Reproduced with permission of the SBMR.)

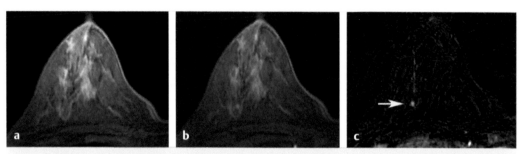

Fig. 7.1 Utility of subtraction images for magnetic resonance imaging interpretation. Assessment for enhancement by comparing the axial precontrast (**a**) and postcontrast (**b**) fat-saturated T1-weighted images may be difficult. A focus of enhancement is more readily apparent when the two images are subtracted (**c**, *arrow*). Subtraction images facilitate initial identification for areas of enhancement. However, once identified, the postcontrast source images should be used to assess lesion morphology.

7.3.1 Background Parenchymal Enhancement

Once the amount of FGT has been assessed, the next step in MR interpretation is to assess the level of the BPE. BPE refers to the amount and degree of enhancement of the normal breast parenchyma. The BI-RADS recommends that each MRI report contains a description of the level of BPE. BPE is classified as minimal (< 25% of glandular tissue demonstrating enhancement), mild (25 to < 50% enhancement), moderate (50 to < 75% enhancement), or marked (> 75% enhancement). The level

of BPE does not correlate with the amount of FGT. Therefore, a breast with extreme fibroglandular tissue may demonstrate minimal BPE and a breast composed of scattered fibroglandular tissue may have moderate or marked BPE.[5] Early studies have suggested that BPE is a marker of breast cancer risk, with the odds of breast cancer increasing with increasing levels of BPE.[6]

Studies have also shown that BPE is hormonally influenced. BPE typically increases during the 4th week of the menstrual cycle and with hormone replacement therapy and lactational change. Similarly, factors known to decrease the degree of BPE include postmenopausal status, antiestrogen therapy (i.e., tamoxifen and aromatase inhibitors) and radiation therapy (▶ Fig. 7.2).[7,8,9,10] BPE may also increase following the cessation of antihormonal therapy. In patients who discontinue tamoxifen, this increase in BPE sometimes is referred to as tamoxifen rebound. Therefore, it is important to know the patient's history when interpreting breast MRI. Factors such as date of the last menstrual period, prior history of radiation therapy, and use of hormonal and antihormonal therapy should be captured at the time of the MRI to facilitate interpretation. Although it is often recommended the screening breast MRIs be performed during the days 7 to 10 of the menstrual cycle to minimize the degree of BPE, more recent studies have suggested that the degree of BPE does not impact the sensitivity or specificity of MR interpretation.

BPE usually demonstrates slow early initial enhancement, and progressive delayed enhancement kinetics.[11] The classic pattern of BPE is sometimes referred to as a "cortical pattern" where there is symmetric preferential enhancement of the peripheral breast parenchyma (▶ Fig. 7.2). However, BPE may also appear scattered foci of enhancement; this was previously referred to as a stippled pattern of nonmass

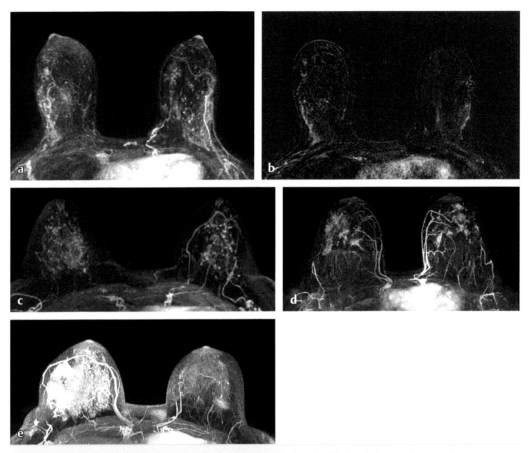

Fig. 7.2 Variations in normal background parenchymal enhancement (BPE). (**a,b**) Axial subtraction maximum intensity projection (MIP) images demonstrate the most classic appearance of BPE where there is preferential enhancement of the peripheral areas of the glandular tissue especially in the upper outer quadrants. This pattern is sometimes referred to as a cortical pattern of enhancement. (**c**) Axial subtraction MIP image demonstrates scattered similar-appearing foci, another common presentation of normal BPE. In the prior Breast Imaging Reporting and Data System (BI-RADS) lexicon, this pattern was described as stippled enhancement. (**d**) Axial subtraction MIP demonstrates bilateral scattered similar-appearing areas of focal NME, also representing a variation of BPE. (**e**) Axial subtraction MIP image demonstrates asymmetric BPE that is marked in the right breast and minimal in the left breast in this patient with a history of left lumpectomy and radiation therapy. Patient history is important when interpreting breast magnetic resonance imaging.

enhancement (NME) in the first edition of the MRI BI-RADS lexicon (▶ Fig. 7.2). The term stippled was removed in the second edition of the lexicon as this pattern is now known to represent normal BPE and not a type of NME.[4] BPE may also present as asymmetric, regional, or focal enhancement. One of the most difficult aspects of breast MR interpretation is distinguishing variations of BPE from abnormal NME.

7.4 Identifying Unique Findings

Once the pattern of BPE has been assessed, the next step is to identify lesions that are unique or distinct from the BPE. The fundamental aspect of AB-MR interpretation is identifying findings that are truly unique to the patient's overall enhancement pattern. Biopsy of findings that are not clearly unique should be minimized in order to maintain high specificity. MIPs and subtraction MIPs are typically generated from the precontrast and first postcontrast series. MIPs are generated using a processing method that projects the pixel with the highest signal onto a projection plane. The MIP and subtraction MIPS provide an overview of the breast, allowing the reader to have a general sense of the level of BPE and whether there is a truly unique finding distinct from the background enhancement that warrants further analysis (▶ Fig. 7.3). Lesion detection at breast MRI is based on identifying lesions with increased vascularity and therefore enhancement relative to normal breast tissue.

Once a unique finding has been identified on the subtraction MIPs and postcontrast images, the enhancing lesion can be classified into one of three general categories: focus, mass, and NME. Characterization of these lesions is based on a combination of lesion morphology on the postcontrast images and the internal signal characteristics on the precontrast T1- and T2-weighted images. While the subtraction series is useful in identifying areas of enhancement, the source images should be used for lesion characterization. Appropriate window and leveling of the postcontrast images are necessary to appreciate a lesion's internal features. When evaluating the T2 signal intensity, it is important to define high T2 signal intensity as signal higher than that of the normal glandular tissue and equivalent to the signal of cyst fluid or normal lymph nodes. The window and level should be adjusted so that differences in signal intensity between fat, tissue, and fluid can be appreciated. If the window and level are set at too narrow of a range, then areas may falsely appear as being bright on T2 images.

7.5 Focus

A focus is historically defined as a dot of enhancement less than 5 mm in size that is too small to further characterize in terms of its margins or internal enhancement pattern due to insufficient spatial resolution or volume averaging. With improved imaging protocols and spatial resolution, one is often able to distinguish between a small < 5 mm mass and a true focus which is a tiny dot of enhancement. Biopsy should not be recommended for foci < 3 mm in size on a baseline study due to the low probability of malignancy in lesions this size particularly in average- and intermediate-risk women.

Multiple scattered foci are almost always a manifestation of normal BPE. Multiple scattered similar-appearing foci are one appearance of BPE and require no additional analysis. In this situation, the AB-MR should be interpreted as normal.

In the past, due to their small size, low predictive value, and the inability to accurately characterize their morphology, a focus detected on breast MRI was routinely disregarded as being either benign or probably benign. Liberman et al found that the frequency of malignancy increased significantly with lesion size. In their cohort of 666 consecutive lesions identified on breast MR images alone, < 1% of all cancers detected were due to a focus and only 3% of foci (lesions < 5 mm in size) represented a malignancy.[12] Similarly, Eby et al reported that foci comprised 46% of BI-RADS 3 lesions and only 1 focus out of 168 was found on follow-up to represent malignancy.[13] Therefore, the majority of foci are benign. However, if a focus of enhancement is unique or distinct from the BPE, then further analysis of the lesion characteristics and morphology is required. Often the subtraction MIP images are useful in putting a potentially unique focus into the context of the normal BPE. If a focus is unique to the background pattern, then further analysis should be performed to determine whether it is benign, probably benign, or suspicious.

On a full MR protocol, enhancement kinetics are not routinely used to characterize a focus. Eby et al reported that the one focus that was found to represent a malignant lesion demonstrated washout kinetics.[13] However, Ha et al subsequently reported that of four malignant foci, two

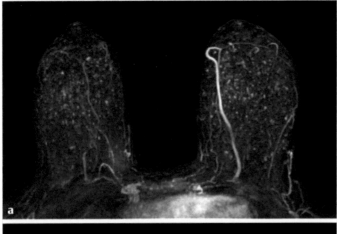

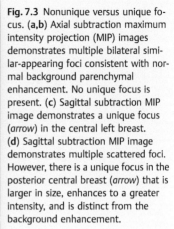

Fig. 7.3 Nonunique versus unique focus. (a,b) Axial subtraction maximum intensity projection (MIP) images demonstrates multiple bilateral similar-appearing foci consistent with normal background parenchymal enhancement. No unique focus is present. (c) Sagittal subtraction MIP image demonstrates a unique focus (*arrow*) in the central left breast. (d) Sagittal subtraction MIP image demonstrates multiple scattered foci. However, there is a unique focus in the posterior central breast (*arrow*) that is larger in size, enhances to a greater intensity, and is distinct from the background enhancement.

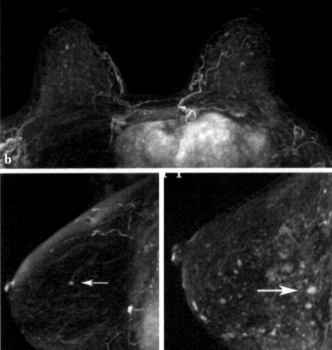

demonstrated benign progressive kinetics and two demonstrated washout kinetics.[14] Evaluation of a

focus should be based on the internal composition and morphology and not on kinetics.

The first step in evaluating a focus is to confirm that it is truly a unique finding and distinct from the BPE. No other similar focus should be present elsewhere in that breast or in the contralateral breast. Once a focus is confirmed to be unique, the next step is to evaluate its morphology (Algorithm 2 (p.91)[2]). The subtraction images are useful in identifying unique findings such as a unique focus, but analysis of the morphology of

---

[2] The Society of Breast MRI Interpretation Guidelines suggest a standardized method for abbreviated breast MRI interpretation. These algorithms are not meant to dictate individual case management decisions. The ultimate decision regarding AB-MR interpretation must be made by the interpreting radiologist in light of all the circumstances presented in an individual examination.

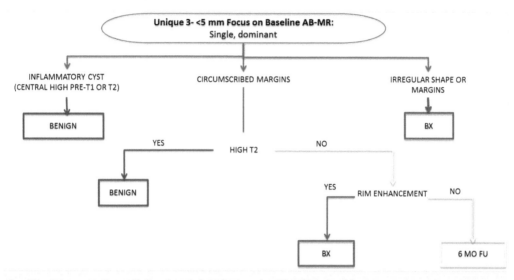

Algorithm 2 Interpretation guidelines for a unique focus on baseline abbreviated breast magnetic resonance imaging (AB-MR). (Reproduced with permission of the SBMR.)

any finding should always be made on the source (i.e., postcontrast T1-weighted) images and not on the subtraction series.

If there is a unique focus, the first step in evaluation is to determine whether it represents a small inflammatory cyst, a unique focus with circumscribed margins, or a unique focus with noncircumscribed margins.

Small inflammatory cysts/cysts with pericystic inflammation have high signal on either the precontrast T1 or the T2 images that match the size and shape of the central dark area on the postcontrast images (▶ Fig. 7.4). Inflammatory cysts are benign and routine follow-up should be recommended.

Any unique focus with an irregular shape or margin requires biopsy (▶ Fig. 7.5). However, as previously mentioned, biopsy should be reserved for a focus ≥ 3 mm in size on a baseline AB-MR.

A unique focus with a circumscribed margin should then be evaluated to determine if there is a high T2 signal intensity correlate. The high T2 signal intensity correlate should also be circumscribed and match the size and shape of the focus. A unique focus on a baseline MRI that is a smooth circumscribed dot of enhancement with a smooth high T2 signal intensity correlate is benign (▶ Fig. 7.6). This characterization of such a focus as benign uses a combination of benign morphology (circumscribed dot of enhancement) and benign intrinsic characteristics (high signal on T2-weighted images).

If there is a unique ≥ 3 mm focus with circumscribed margins and no high T2 signal correlate on a baseline AB-MR, the focus should be evaluated to determine whether rim enhancement is present. Biopsy should be recommended for a circumscribed unique ≥ 3 mm circumscribed, low T2 rim-enhancing focus (▶ Fig. 7.7). The combination of low T2 signal intensity and the presence of rim enhancement are suspicious enough to warrant biopsy.

Algorithm 2 (p.91) applies to a unique ≥ 3 mm focus on a baseline AB-MR. If comparison studies are available, biopsy should be recommended for any discrete unique focus that is new or increasing in size. In addition, the threshold for biopsy of a focus in a patient with a history of lumpectomy and radiation therapy should be lowered especially if that focus is in the treated irradiated breast.

In some cases, there is not a unique single focus but multiple foci. As discussed earlier, multiple bilateral scattered similar-appearing foci represent normal BPE and do not require additional analysis or workup. However, there may be a group of foci that are more concentrated or grouped in one area compared to the background. If these foci are in a linear distribution, then biopsy should be recommended, as this may represent an early area of clumped or linear NME. If this group of foci is not in a linear distribution, then a recommendation for a 6-month follow-up MRI would be appropriate.

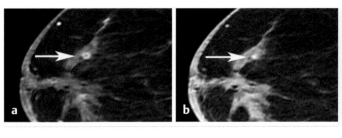

Fig. 7.4 Examples of small inflammatory cyst. Axial postcontrast fat-saturated T1-weighted image demonstrates a rim-enhancing focus (**a**, *arrow*) with a corresponding central dot of high signal intensity on the precontrast images (**b**, *arrow*) consistent with a proteinaceous cyst.

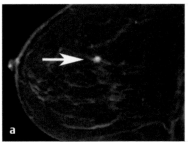
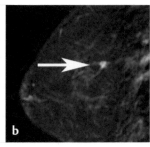

Fig. 7.5 Examples of suspicious foci. (**a**) Sagittal subtraction demonstrates a 4-mm focus with irregular margins (*arrow*). (**b**) Sagittal postcontrast fat-saturated T1-weighted image demonstrates another example of a focus with an irregular margin (*arrow*).

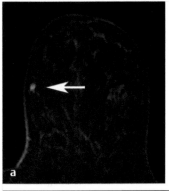
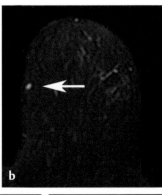
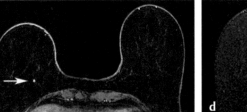

Fig. 7.6 Benign versus probably benign focus. Axial postcontrast fat-saturated T1-weighted image demonstrates a unique rim-enhancing focus with smooth circumscribed margins (**a**, *arrow*) and a high T2 signal intensity correlate (**b**, *arrow*). A circumscribed unique focus with a high T2 correlate is almost always benign and routine screening should be recommended. Axial postcontrast T1-weighted image demonstrates a unique focus with smooth circumscribed margins (**c**, *arrow*) and no high T2 correlate (**d**). A 6-month follow-up is appropriate for a circumscribed focus and no high T2 correlate.

7.6 Mass

A mass is defined as a space-occupying lesion ≥ 5 mm in size and usually has a correlate on precontrast T1- or T2-weighted images.[4] As described in the second edition of the American College of Radiology BI-RADS lexicon, a mass should be characterized by its shape, margins, and internal enhancement pattern. The shape of a mass may be round, oval (which includes lobulated), or irregular; the margins may be circumscribed or not circumscribed (spiculated or irregular).[4] Internal enhancement pattern should be described as having homogeneous, heterogeneous, or rim enhancement, or as having dark internal septations.[4] On AB-MR, these same features are assessed to determine whether a mass is benign (BI-RADS 2), probably benign (BI-RADS 3), or suspicious (BI-RADS 4)/highly suspicious (BI-RADS 5).

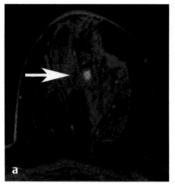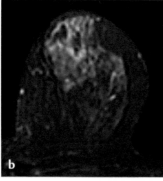

Fig. 7.7 Rim-enhancing focus. (**a**) Axial postcontrast fat-saturated T1-weighted image demonstrates a unique rim-enhancing focus (*arrow*) with no correlate on the precontrast T2-weighted image (**b**). Biopsy yielded infiltrating ductal carcinoma.

Lesion morphology is the primary feature used in assessing masses. Imaging features of masses that are most suggestive of malignancy include spiculated or irregular margins and rim enhancement. Schnall et al reported that margin description was the single feature of masses most predictive of malignancy.[3] Rim enhancement was also highly predictive of malignancy, but not frequently present. Gutierrez et al found that of 123 suspicious masses, size of ≥ 1 cm, lobular or irregular shape, irregular or spiculated margins, and heterogeneous or rim enhancement were associated with higher odds of malignancy.[15] Masses ≥ 1 cm in size with heterogeneous enhancement and irregular margins had a 68% probability of malignancy.

The primary difference between interpretation of an AB-MR and a full MR protocol with only one postcontrast series is that delayed kinetic information cannot be used to determine management of an area of enhancement. However, MR interpretation has always relied primarily on lesion morphology and internal composition (fat or fluid content on the T1- and T2-weighted sequences), given there is considerable overlap in the kinetic patterns of benign and malignant lesions. Although invasive cancers classically demonstrate intense early enhancement and rapid washout, some malignant lesions display benign kinetic patterns and some benign lesions displaying delayed washout kinetics.[3,16,17] Bluemke et al reported that in 209 patients with ductal carcinomas in situ (DCIS) or invasive cancer, a washout kinetic pattern was present in 43, resulting in a sensitivity of 20.5%.[17] Schnall et al reported that although a mass demonstrating washout kinetics was five times more likely to represent a malignant lesion, 45% of cancers in their study demonstrated

a persistent enhancement pattern.[3] Also, many benign masses, including lymph nodes and papillomas may demonstrate suspicious washout kinetics. Therefore, the loss of kinetic information with an abbreviated protocol using only a single postcontrast series should not significantly impact sensitivity, and interpretation should be based on the morphology and composition of the mass.[3,18] The lack of kinetic information could reduce sensitivity of cancers with completely benign morphology that are only detected due to suspicious washout kinetics. However, this is extremely uncommon. Careful morphological analysis should maintain high sensitivity with AB-MR.

7.7 Approach to Unique Mass

The following section will discuss a general approach to evaluating a unique mass on a baseline AB-MR (Algorithm 3 (p.93) [3]). The first step is to determine whether this represents a classically benign mass, such as an inflammatory cyst, degenerated fibroadenoma, or classic lymph node. It is important to avoid biopsy or follow up on classically benign masses. Classically benign masses on MRI included inflammatory cysts, intramammary lymph nodes, degenerated fibroadenomas, and fat necrosis.

---

[3] The Society of Breast MRI Interpretation Guidelines suggest a standardized method for abbreviated breast MRI interpretation. These algorithms are not meant to dictate individual case management decisions. The ultimate decision regarding AB-MR interpretation must be made by the interpreting radiologist in light of all the circumstances presented in an individual examination.

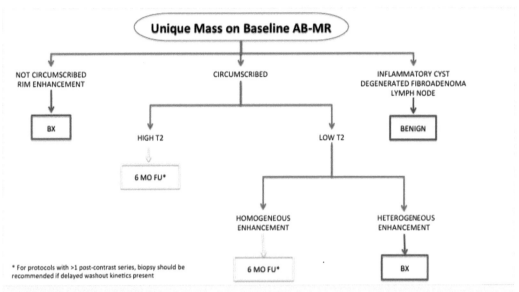

Algorithm 3 Interpretation guidelines for a unique mass on baseline abbreviated breast magnetic resonance imaging. (Reproduced with permission of the SBMR.)

7.7.1 Classically Benign Masses

Inflammatory Cysts

Cysts are circumscribed mass that are high on T2- or T1-weighted precontrast images if they contain proteinaceous or hemorrhagic debris. Cysts do not enhance, but may be associated with pericystic inflammation, thought to be due to compression of the adjacent tissue or leakage of fluid causing reactive inflammation or fibrosis. Pericystic inflammation or inflammatory cysts are commonly referred to as having the solar eclipse sign. On both postcontrast and subtraction images, there is a smooth interface between the surrounding inflammation and the cyst which appears dark on the subtraction images (▶ Fig. 7.8). The dark central cavity on the subtraction image should match in size with the cyst on the T2 or precontrast T1-weighted images.

Pericystic inflammation must be distinguished from a rim-enhancing mass. With a rim-enhancing mass, the peripheral enhancement is not in the adjacent surrounding tissue as with pericystic inflammation but within the mass itself. Rim-enhancing masses may also have a high signal correlate on the T2 or precontrast T1-weighted images. However, the area that is bright on the T2 or precontrast T1-weighted images will not match the dark center of the rim-enhancing mass on the subtraction images, as it would with an inflammatory cyst. The peripheral enhancement may be either within or larger than the area that has high signal on the T2 or precontrast T1-weighted images (▶ Fig. 7.9). Therefore, careful correlation should be made to compare the size and shape of the dark central cavity of a peripherally enhancing mass on the subtraction with the correlate on the precontrast T1- or T2-weighted images to distinguish an inflammatory cyst from a rim-enhancing mass. In addition, rim-enhancing high T1- or T2-weighted masses have irregular internal and external walls, in contrast to the smooth inner edge representing the interface between the cyst and the surrounding enhancing tissue (▶ Fig. 7.9). Rim-enhancing masses also may be low signal on the precontrast T1- and T2-weighted images.

Breast cancers may rarely present as high T2 signal intensity masses. Careful analysis of lesion morphology usually reveals suspicious morphological features despite the seemingly benign high T2 signal. Mucinous cancers are typically homogeneously high signal on T2-weighted images due to their mucin content. However, mucinous cancers usually demonstrate heterogeneous or rim enhancement and irregular margins. Papillary cancers also may demonstrate high T2 signal intensity, but like mucinous cancers are easily distinguished from inflammatory cysts or benign masses by their internal enhancement pattern

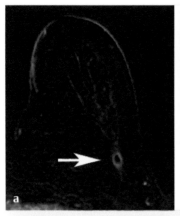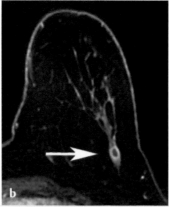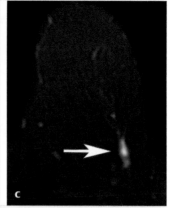

Fig. 7.8 Inflammatory cyst. Axial subtraction (**a**, *arrow*) and postcontrast fat-saturated T1-weighted (**b**, *arrow*) images demonstrate a peripherally enhancing mass (*arrow*). A high T2 signal intensity cyst (**c**, *arrow*) is seen on the axial postcontrast fat-saturated T2-weighted image that matches in size and shape to the dark central cavity on the postcontrast image; findings represent an inflammatory cyst.

and/or margins. Triple negative cancers may present as circumscribed, high T2 signal intensity masses but are relatively uncommon. Therefore, a 6-month follow-up MRI should be recommended for a circumscribed, high T2 signal intensity homogeneously or heterogeneously enhancing mass to confirm benignity.

Lymph Nodes

Lymph nodes are circumscribed lobulated masses that are typically high on T2-weighted images and are usually located superficially in the upper outer quadrant and commonly adjacent to blood vessels (▶ Fig. 7.10). On a standard MRI protocol, lymph nodes classically demonstrate delayed washout kinetics, and represent an example of a benign mass displaying a suspicious enhancement pattern. In an AB-MR protocol, lymph nodes can be accurately characterized using the combination of morphology, T2 signal intensity, hilar cleft, and location.

Degenerated Fibroadenoma

The classic appearance of a fibroadenoma is a circumscribed, homogeneously high T2 signal intensity round or lobulated mass with dark internal septations and progressive enhancement kinetics. As discussed below, a BI-RADS 3 recommendation is appropriate for a classic fibroadenoma. More commonly, fibroadenomas are degenerated or sclerosed, presenting as circumscribed masses with low or intermediate T2 signal, low-level internal enhancement (i.e., incomplete enhancement at > 50% threshold) with or without dark internal septations (▶ Fig. 7.11). A degenerating or sclerosed fibroadenoma with low-level enhancement is benign and should be given a BI-RADS 2 recommendation.

Postsurgical Change and Fat Necrosis

Postsurgical change may present as areas of distortion with low-level cloudy enhancement, seromas with smooth, thin rim enhancement, or areas of fat necrosis. Fat necrosis commonly demonstrates washout kinetics and is another example of a benign etiology that typically displays a suspicious enhancement pattern. The loss of delayed kinetics with an AB-MR protocol using only one postcontrast series should not impact characterization of areas of fat necrosis. On AB-MR, fat necrosis may be seen in areas of postsurgical change or trauma and will appear as areas of peripheral enhancement with internal signal similar to other areas of fat in the breast. Fat necrosis may also present as areas of low-level NME that is concentric around a postsurgical scar.

7.7.2 Mass Margins and Rim Enhancement

Once classically benign masses are excluded, the next step in assessing a unique mass on a baseline AB-MR is to evaluate the mass margins and

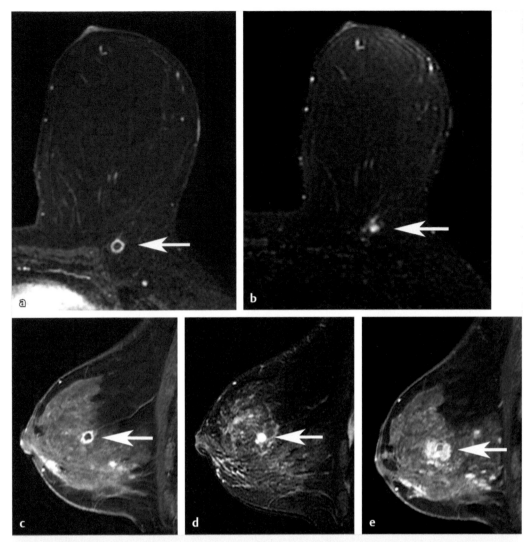

Fig. 7.9 Examples of rim-enhancing masses. (**a**) Axial postcontrast T1-weighted fat-saturated image demonstrate a rim-enhancing mass (*arrow*). (**b**) An area of high signal is seen on the T2-weighted fat-saturated image (*arrow*). However, the area of high signal on the T2-weighted image does not match in size and shape to the dark central area on the postcontrast fat-saturated T1 weighted image and fat-saturated T2-weighted image. These findings are consistent with a rim-enhancing mass and not an inflammatory cyst. Biopsy yielded invasive ductal carcinoma. (**c**) Sagittal postcontrast T1-weighted image demonstrates a rim-enhancing mass with an irregular internal wall (*arrow*). (**d**) A high T2 signal intensity correlate matching the central cavity is present (*arrow*). However, the irregularity of the inner wall should prompt biopsy, which is distinguishable from the smooth inner wall seen with inflammatory cysts. (**e**) Magnetic resonance imaging performed 6 months later demonstrates increase in size (*arrow*). Biopsy yielded invasive ductal carcinoma. These examples demonstrate the importance of distinguishing benign inflammatory cysts from rim-enhancing cancers.

the presence of rim enhancement. The margins of a mass are either circumscribed or noncircumscribed (▶ Fig. 7.12). The entire margin must be well defined for the margin to be considered circumscribed. With rim enhancement, there is increased enhancement at the periphery of the mass. Noncircumscribed margins or rim enhancement are strongly suggestive of malignancy, and the presence of these should prompt a recommendation for biopsy (▶ Fig. 7.13). For example, the

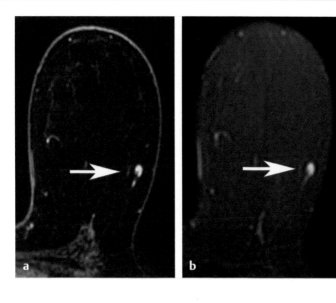

Fig. 7.10 Classically benign mass: intramammary lymph node. An intramammary node classically appears as circumscribed lobulated mass with a hilar cleft on the postcontrast T1-weighted image (**a**, *arrow*) and has a high T2 signal intensity correlate (**b**, *arrow*). Intramammary nodes are often superficially located in the upper outer quadrants and adjacent to blood vessels.

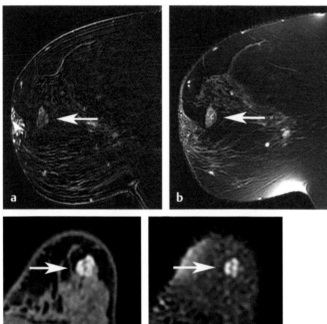

Fig. 7.11 Varying appearances of fibroadenomas. Sagittal postcontrast T1-weighted image demonstrates a circumscribed mass with low-level enhancement (**a**, *arrow*) or incomplete enhancement at 50% threshold and low signal on the T2-weighted fat-saturated image (**b**, *arrow*). Imaging appearance is characteristic of a degenerated fibroadenoma, which is a classically benign mass that requires no additional follow-up. Axial postcontrast T1-weighted fat-saturated image demonstrates a circumscribed homogeneously enhancing mass with dark internal septations (**c**) and a high signal intensity correlate on the corresponding T2-weighted image (**d**). These are the imaging features of a classic fibroadenoma; a 6-month follow-up is appropriate for a solitary probable fibroadenoma on baseline abbreviated breast magnetic resonance imaging.

positive predictive value (PPV3) of spiculated margins has been reported to be as high as 76 to 88%, while that of rim enhancement is 76 to 88%. Therefore, biopsy should be recommended for any solitary mass that is not circumscribed or that demonstrates rim internal enhancement, regardless of the enhancement kinetic pattern.

7.7.3 T2 Signal Intensity

If a unique mass is circumscribed and does not demonstrate rim enhancement, further management will depend on the signal intensity on the T2-weighted images and internal enhancement pattern. Attention should be paid to appropriately

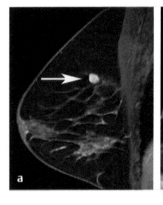
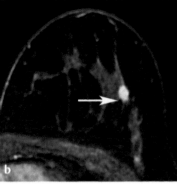

Fig. 7.12 Circumscribed versus noncircumscribed mass margins. The margins of a mass are circumscribed (**a**, *arrow*) or noncircumscribed (**b**). The entire margin must be well defined for the margin to be considered circumscribed. If any portion is ill defined (**b**, *arrow*), the mass should be considered noncircumscribed.

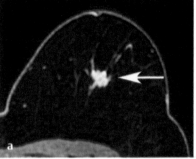
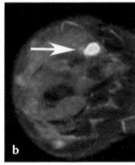

Fig. 7.13 Classic appearances of malignant masses. Suspicious morphological features of masses include noncircumscribed margins and rim enhancement. Postcontrast T1-weighted fat-saturated image demonstrates an irregular noncircumscribed mass (**a**, *arrow*) and a rim-enhancing mass (**b**, *arrow*). Biopsy should be recommended for any irregular or rim-enhancing mass.

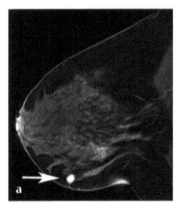
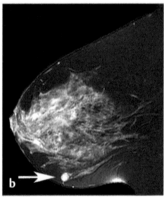

Fig. 7.14 Probably benign high T2 circumscribed mass. Sagittal postcontrast T1-weighted fat-saturated image demonstrates a circumscribed mass with dark internal septations (**a**, arrow) and a high T2 signal correlate (**b**, *arrow*), probably representing a fibroadenoma. A BI-RADS 3 recommendation would be appropriate.

set the window and level so that cysts and vessels are bright but not oversaturated on the T2-weighted sequence. High T2 signal masses on MRI have signal intensity higher than the glandular tissue and equivalent to cysts or vessels. Circumscribed masses that are high signal on T2-weighted images with either homogeneous or heterogeneous internal enhancement are probably benign (▶ Fig. 7.14). A 6-month follow-up is appropriate for a circumscribed, high T2 signal intensity homogeneously or heterogeneously enhancing mass seen on a baseline MRI in the average- or intermediate-risk patient due to the combination of benign morphology, internal composition, and enhancement pattern (i.e., not rim enhancing). Breast cancers that are high signal on T2-weighted images are unusual unless rim enhancement or irregular margins are present. However, if the AB-MR protocol includes more than one postcontrast series, biopsy should be recommended if the circumscribed high T2 homogeneously or heterogeneously enhancing mass demonstrates washout kinetics.

A high T2 signal intensity, circumscribed mass may represent a fibroadenoma. The classic imaging features of a fibroadenoma is a circumscribed, homogeneously high T2 signal intensity round or lobulated mass with dark internal septations and progressive enhancement kinetics (▶ Fig. 7.14). On AB-MR, a BI-RADS 3 recommendation would be appropriate for a probable fibroadenoma on a baseline study.

However, dark internal septations may also be seen in malignant lesions, and a single morphologic feature should not be used to characterize a mass. Schnall et at reported that nonenhancing internal septations were found in 47% of enhancing masses representing cancer.[3] Therefore, the presence of dark internal septations is only reassuring of a benign or probably benign lesion if the mass also has circumscribed margins and otherwise homogeneous enhancement. Biopsy should be recommended for an oval mass with noncircumscribed margins, high T2 signal intensity, and dark internal septations. Similar to mammography, ultrasound, and conventional breast MRI, characterization of a mass on AB-MR should be based primarily on the most suspicious morphological feature. Correlation with mammography or prior ultrasounds is also important. If long-term stability of the enhancing mass can be demonstrated on prior mammograms or ultrasound, then the BI-RADS 3 recommendation may be downgraded to a BI-RADS 2 recommendation, with no additional workup or follow-up needed.

7.7.4 Low T2 SI Mass and Internal Enhancement Pattern: Homogeneous versus Heterogeneous

For enhancing low or intermediate T2 signal intensity circumscribed masses, management will depend on the internal enhancement pattern. A BI-RADS 3 recommendation is appropriate for a homogeneously enhancing low or intermediate T2 signal intensity circumscribed mass (▶ Fig. 7.15). However, if > 1 postcontrast series are obtained and the circumscribed intermediate or low T2 homogeneously enhancing mass demonstrates washout kinetics, biopsy should be recommended.

Biopsy should also be recommended for a unique circumscribed, low or intermediate T2 signal mass with heterogeneous enhancement because both the internal composition (not high T2) and enhancement pattern (not homogeneously enhancing) are not alone characteristic of a benign mass (▶ Fig. 7.15). When these two features are seen together, the probability of malignancy is sufficient enough to recommend biopsy.

7.8 Multiple Masses

Similar to mammography, a BI-RADS 2 recommendation is appropriate when there are multiple bilateral similar-appearing circumscribed masses. In the situation of multiple similar benign appearing circumscribed masses that are unilateral, a 6-month follow-up may be appropriate. If there are multiple similar-appearing masses and

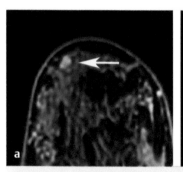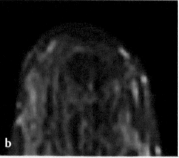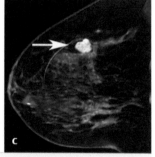

Fig. 7.15 Low or intermediate T2 circumscribed masses. Management of a low or intermediate T2 circumscribed mass will depend on the internal enhancement pattern. Axial postcontrast T1-weighted fat-saturated image demonstrates a circumscribed homogeneously enhancing mass with dark internal septations (**a**, *arrow*) and no high T2 correlate (**b**). A 6-month follow-up would be appropriate. Sagittal postcontrast T1-weighted fat-saturated image demonstrates a circumscribed mass with heterogeneous enhancement (**c**, *arrow*) and no high T2 correlate. The combination of a low T2 signal and heterogeneous internal enhancement should prompt a recommendation for biopsy despite the circumscribed margins.

one appears suspicious and different in morphology, internal composition, or enhancement pattern from the others, then biopsy of that unique mass should be recommended. Biopsy of a representative mass should also be recommended if there are multiple suspicious noncircumscribed masses.

Finally, the above interpretation guidelines apply to a mass or multiple masses seen on a baseline AB-MR. Any mass that is new or enlarging on a subsequent screening or follow-up MRI requires biopsy to obtain a pathological diagnosis, even if the morphological features appear benign.

7.9 Approach to Unique Nonmass Enhancement

This section will discuss an approach to evaluating a unique area of NME (Algorithm 4 (p. 100) [4]).

NME refers to an area of enhancement that appears distinct from the normal breast parenchyma. NME occurs in an area of the fibroglandular tissue that otherwise appears normal on precontrast images. There is no space-occupying effect; the enhancing area usually has no correlate on fat-suppressed or non–fat-suppressed T1-weighted images.

7.9.1 Nonmass Enhancement: Distribution

Areas of NME should be characterized using descriptors as outlined in the BI-RADS atlas. The lexicon describes areas of NME in terms of their distribution (focal, linear, segmental, regional, multiple regions, or diffuse) and internal enhancement pattern (homogeneous, heterogeneous, clumped, or clustered ring).[4] The term "stippled" was removed in the BI-RADS atlas as scattered foci of enhancement are now known to represent a manifestation of normal BPE.

A focal distribution refers to NME in a confined area occupying less than a quadrant. Linear NME is enhancement in a line, suggesting enhancement within a duct or its branches. A segmental distribution involves a triangular area

with the apex pointing toward the nipple. Regional NME occupies at last a quadrant of a breast, while multiple regions involve at least two large separate volumes of tissue not conforming to a ductal distribution. Diffuse NME is enhancement distributed randomly throughout the breast.[4]

7.9.2 Nonmass Enhancement: Internal Enhancement Pattern

NME is also characterized by the internal enhancement pattern. Homogeneous describes uniform internal enhancement, while heterogeneous is used to describe internal enhancement that is not uniform and separated by normal glandular tissue or fat. Clumped NME refers to enhancement in a cobblestone or beaded pattern that may be confluent in areas. Finally, the clustered ring pattern refers to thin rings of enhancement clustered around ducts.[4]

Most causes of NME are benign, and include focal or diffuse fibrocystic change, adenosis, and stromal fibrosis. However, DCIS and invasive lobular carcinoma commonly present as areas of NME. DCIS in particular classically appears as NME in a linear or segmental distribution with clumped or heterogeneous internal enhancement.

Similar to descriptors used for enhancing masses, multiple studies have correlated BI-RADS descriptors for NME and the likelihood of malignancy. Some studies have found that certain NME descriptors are suggestive of malignancy. In a small retrospective study, Liberman et al reported that segmental (67% carcinoma) or clumped linear or ductal NME (31% carcinoma) had the highest PPV for malignancy.[19] Schnall et al reported that NME in a ductal distribution was associated with a 59% likelihood of malignancy, while 78% of areas of segmental NME represented cancer.[3] More recently, Mahoney et al found that linear NME (17%) and ductal NME (50%) were the distribution descriptors with the highest PPVs for malignancy, and that clumped NME (30%) was the internal enhancement descriptor most likely to represent malignancy.[18]

However, other studies have suggested that BI-RADS descriptors of morphology and internal enhancement patterns for NME are unreliable in predicting the likelihood of malignancy. Gutierrez et al found that BI-RADS descriptors were useful in predicting the likelihood of malignancy for enhancing masses, but not areas of NME.[15] Baltzer

---

[4] The Society of Breast MRI Interpretation Guidelines suggest a standardized method for abbreviated breast MRI interpretation. These algorithms are not meant to dictate individual case management decisions. The ultimate decision regarding AB-MR interpretation must be made by the interpreting radiologist in light of all the circumstances presented in an individual examination.

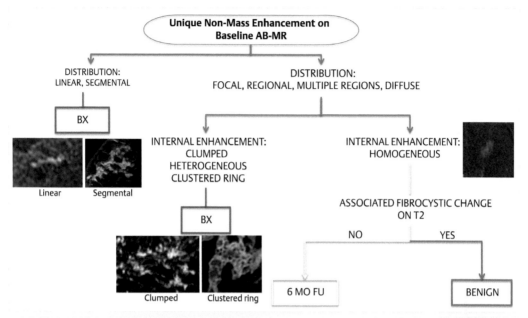

Algorithm 4 Interpretation guidelines for unique nonmass enhancement on baseline abbreviated breast magnetic resonance imaging. (Reproduced with permission of the SBMR.)

et al similarly reported that areas of NME were a frequent cause of false positives on breast MRI and that BI-RADS descriptors were not sufficient for differentiating benign and malignant NME.[20] These conflicting results may partly be due to the suboptimal agreement among radiologists in using the descriptors to characterize areas of NME.

Most studies evaluating the utility of BI-RADS descriptors are also limited by the fact that the BI-RADS descriptors for distribution and internal enhancement patterns were evaluated individually and not in combination. In reality, a combination of these features is used in determining a final assessment.

Multiple studies have evaluated the role of kinetic information in distinguishing benign from malignant causes of NME. Both DCIS and invasive lobular carcinoma (ILC) may demonstrate benign enhancement kinetic patterns such as slow early enhancement and persistent delayed enhancement. Therefore, similar to the evaluation of enhancing masses, lesion morphology, and not enhancement kinetics, should be the primary determinant in characterizing an area of NME.[3,18] As DCIS and ILC do not infrequently demonstrate

persistent delayed enhancement, the loss of delayed enhancement kinetics with an AB-MR protocol should not impact sensitivity for breast cancer detection.

The art of breast MRI is distinguishing variations of normal BPE from areas of NME. As discussed, the classic appearance of BPE is diffuse symmetric areas of enhancement, but BPE may appear as asymmetric focal or regional areas of enhancement that may be difficult to distinguish from NME.

A unique area of NME should first be characterized by its distribution. Any unique NMC in a linear or segmental distribution requires biopsy due to the high PPV for malignancy (▶ Fig. 7.16). The PPV for regional enhancement varies widely in the literature. For example, Mahoney et al reported a PPV of 4%, while Schnall et al found that regional enhancement was associated with malignancy in 21%.[3,18] Multiple regions and diffuse NME are often benign, but can represent extensive areas of malignancy (▶ Fig. 7.16).

Therefore, the next step in the assessment of focal, regional, multiple regions, or diffuse NME is

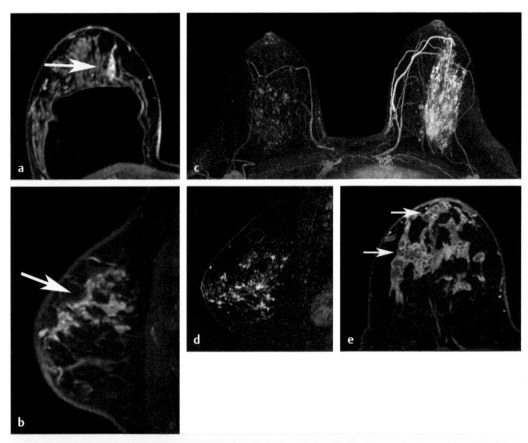

Fig. 7.16 Suspicious nonmass enhancement (NME). Axial postcontrast T1-weighted image demonstrates an area of clumped linear NME (**a**, *arrow*) which has a cobblestone pattern extending anteriorly from the implant. Biopsy yielded ductal carcinomas in situ (DCIS). Sagittal postcontrast T1-weighted fat-saturated image (**b**, *arrow*) demonstrates segmental NME in a cone shape with the apex toward the nipple. Biopsy yielded DCIS. Axial subtraction maximum intensity projection image (**c**) demonstrates markedly asymmetric NME in the lateral left breast. Sagittal (**d**) postcontrast T1-weighted image demonstrates clumped and heterogeneous NME involving a multiregional distribution. Biopsy yielded IDC and DCIS. Axial (**e**, *arrows*) postcontrast T1-weighted fat-saturated image demonstrates clustered ring NME. Biopsy yielded DCIS.

to characterize the internal enhancement pattern. NME with a heterogeneous, clumped, or clustered ring pattern of enhancement should be biopsied due to the likelihood of these areas representing cancer (▶ Fig. 7.16 d, e). Therefore, only NME with homogeneous internal enhancement does not require biopsy.

For areas of focal, regional, multiple regions, and diffuse NME with homogeneous internal enhancement, management is based on whether there is corresponding high signal intensity on the T2-weighted images suggesting associated fibrocystic change. If a corresponding high T2 correlate is seen, then a BI-RADS 2 assessment would be appropriate. If there is no high T2 correlate, a 6-month follow-up recommendation is appropriate for homogeneous internal enhancement in a focal, regional, multiregional, or diffuse distribution (▶ Fig. 7.17).

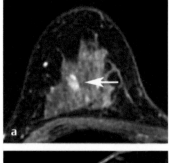

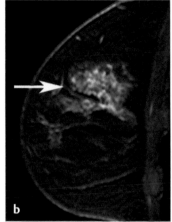

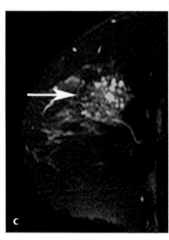

Fig. 7.17 Probably benign versus benign nonmass enhancement (NME). (a) Axial postcontrast T1-weighted image demonstrates an area of focal homogeneous enhancement (*arrow*). No high signal correlate was seen on the T2-weighted images. Therefore, a 6-month follow-up recommendation would be appropriate. (b) Axial postcontrast T1-weighted image demonstrates a focal area of homogeneous nonmass enhancement (*arrow*). (c) A high signal correlate (*arrow*) is seen on the fat-saturated T2-weighted image.

7.10 Conclusion

The basic principles of interpretation of MRIs using an abbreviated protocol are similar to that of a full protocol. In both studies, lesion characterization should primarily be based on lesion morphology and internal composition. Lesion kinetics play a secondary role with standard full protocol MRIs, and are not incorporated with an abbreviated protocol if only a single postcontrast series is acquired. The absence of kinetics most likely will not impact sensitivity, but may result in reduced specificity or increased recommendations for a 6-month follow-up. Using the guidelines provided in this chapter, the goal of AB-MR interpretation would be to maintain the high sensitivity seen with a full MR protocol, with only a slight reduced specificity and recall rate.

References

[1] Schneider BP, Miller KD. Angiogenesis of breast cancer. J Clin Oncol. 2005; 23(8):1782–1790

[2] Weidner N, Semple JP, Welch WR, Folkman J. Tumor angiogenesis and metastasis–correlation in invasive breast carcinoma. N Engl J Med. 1991; 324(1):1–8

[3] Schnall MD, Blume J, Bluemke DA, et al. Diagnostic architectural and dynamic features at breast MR imaging: multicenter study. Radiology. 2006; 238(1):42–53

[4] Morris EA, Comstock CC, Lee CH, et al. ACR BI-RADS® Magnetic Resonance Imaging. In: ACR BI-RADS® Atlas, Breast Imaging Reporting and Data System. Reston, VA: American College of Radiology; 2013

[5] Kuhl C. The current status of breast MR imaging. Part I. Choice of technique, image interpretation, diagnostic accuracy, and transfer to clinical practice. Radiology. 2007; 244 (2):356–378

[6] King V, Brooks JD, Bernstein JL, Reiner AS, Pike MC, Morris EA. Background parenchymal enhancement at breast MR imaging and breast cancer risk. Radiology. 2011; 260(1):50–60

[7] King V, Goldfarb SB, Brooks JD, et al. Effect of aromatase inhibitors on background parenchymal enhancement and amount of fibroglandular tissue at breast MR imaging. Radiology. 2012; 264(3):670–678

[8] King V, Gu Y, Kaplan JB, Brooks JD, Pike MC, Morris EA. Impact of menopausal status on background parenchymal enhancement and fibroglandular tissue on breast MRI. Eur Radiol. 2012; 22(12):2641–2647

[9] King V, Kaplan J, Pike MC, et al. Impact of tamoxifen on amount of fibroglandular tissue, background parenchymal enhancement, and cysts on breast magnetic resonance imaging. Breast J. 2012; 18(6):527–534

[10] Schrading S, Schild H, Kühr M, Kuhl C. Effects of tamoxifen and aromatase inhibitors on breast tissue enhancement in dynamic contrast-enhanced breast MR imaging: a longitudinal intraindividual cohort study. Radiology. 2014; 271 (1):45–55

[11] Giess CS, Yeh ED, Raza S, Birdwell RL. Background parenchymal enhancement at breast MR imaging: normal patterns, diagnostic challenges, and potential for false-positive and false-negative interpretation. Radiographics. 2014; 34(1):234–247

[12] Liberman L, Mason G, Morris EA, Dershaw DD. Does size matter? Positive predictive value of MRI-detected breast lesions as a function of lesion size. AJR Am J Roentgenol. 2006; 186(2):426–430

[13] Eby PR, DeMartini WB, Gutierrez RL, Saini MH, Peacock S, Lehman CD. Characteristics of probably benign breast MRI lesions. AJR Am J Roentgenol. 2009; 193(3):861–867

[14] Ha R, Sung J, Lee C, Comstock C, Wynn R, Morris E. Characteristics and outcome of enhancing foci followed on breast MRI with management implications. Clin Radiol. 2014; 69(7):715–720

[15] Gutierrez RL, DeMartini WB, Eby PR, Kurland BF, Peacock S, Lehman CD. BI-RADS lesion characteristics predict likelihood of malignancy in breast MRI for masses but not for nonmasslike enhancement. AJR Am J Roentgenol. 2009; 193(4):994–1000

[16] Kuhl CK, Mielcareck P, Klaschik S, et al. Dynamic breast MR imaging: are signal intensity time course data useful for differential diagnosis of enhancing lesions? Radiology. 1999; 211(1):101–110

[17] Bluemke DA, Gatsonis CA, Chen MH, et al. Magnetic resonance imaging of the breast prior to biopsy. JAMA. 2004; 292(22):2735–2742

[18] Mahoney MC, Gatsonis C, Hanna L, DeMartini WB, Lehman C. Positive predictive value of BI-RADS MR imaging. Radiology. 2012; 264(1):51–58

[19] Liberman L, Morris EA, Lee MJ, et al. Breast lesions detected on MR imaging: features and positive predictive value. AJR Am J Roentgenol. 2002; 179(1):171–178

[20] Baltzer PA, Benndorf M, Dietzel M, Gajda M, Runnebaum IB, Kaiser WA. False-positive findings at contrast-enhanced breast MRI: a BI-RADS descriptor study. AJR Am J Roentgenol. 2010; 194(6):1658–1663

8 Magnetic Resonance Imaging–Guided Biopsy Techniques

Carol H. Lee

8.1 Introduction

The objective of screening with magnetic resonance imaging (MRI) is to find cancers that are not detected by other imaging modalities or by physical examination. Therefore, it is essential that any facility that does breast MRI, particularly for screening where patients are asymptomatic, has the ability to perform biopsy with MRI guidance. The equipment needed for MRI-guided biopsy is readily available and equipment cost is relatively low compared to the cost of the magnet and coil. In addition, the Medicare Act of 2011 requires that in order to receive reimbursement, outpatient facilities that perform breast MRI must be accredited by an approved accrediting body, one of which is the American College of Radiology (ACR). One of the requirements of ACR MRI accreditation is the ability to perform MRI-guided biopsy. If biopsy is not offered, the facility must have a formal referral relationship with another facility that will accept their patients without the need to repeat the examination in order to become accredited.[1]

Several studies on experience with MRI-guided biopsies have reported a yield of malignancy ranging from 18 to 61%, with most at approximately 25%.[2,3,4,5,6,7,8,9] It has been shown that the positive predictive value (PPV) for malignancy is higher for lesions found on diagnostic exams than on screening studies and the highest PPV occurs in cases in which the biopsied lesion is in a breast with a current ipsilateral cancer. In one study, the PPV of lesions from diagnostic studies was 35% compared to 14% for screening cases, while it was 43% for lesions in breasts with a separate site of known malignancy.[7] Manion et al had a similar experience with a PPV of 16% among the cases done for high-risk screening and 31% in women with a current ipsilateral or contralateral cancer.[9] Therefore, for lesions found on abbreviated breast MRI (AB-MR), the PPV will likely be at the lower end of the range of reported PPVs. ▶ Table 8.1 presents the yield of malignancy in a number of studies of MRI-guided biopsies.

8.2 Targeted Ultrasound

The proportion of cases that require MRI-guided biopsy will vary according to the patient

Table 8.1 Positive predictive value for malignancy at MRI-guided core biopsy

Author (year)	No. of lesions	Needle gauge	Cancers
Perlet et al (2002)[2]	334	11	84 (25%)
Orel et al (2006)[3]	85	9	52 (61%)
Liberman et al (2007)[29]	98	9	24 (25%)
Perlet et al (2006)[5]	517	11	138 (27%)
Mahoney (2008)[6]	55	10	10 (18%)
Han et al (2008)[7]	150	9 or 10	43 (29%)
Rauch et al (2012)[8]	218	9	138 (27%)
Manion et al (2014)[9]	445	Not stated	94 (21%)

population being screened, whether exams are largely prevalence or incidence exams, and the interpretation criteria. When a suspicious finding is seen on breast MRI, a recent mammogram should be reviewed to determine if a possible mammographic correlate is present. Occasionally, faint calcifications or a subtle asymmetry can be seen in retrospect that will allow a stereotactic biopsy to be done for the MR finding. If the mammogram is negative, targeted ultrasound can be performed in an attempt to find a sonographic correlate and perform the biopsy under ultrasound guidance, even if a preceding survey ultrasound was negative. Ultrasound-guided biopsies have a number of advantages over MRI-guided biopsies including being faster, more comfortable, and less expensive.

A number of studies have evaluated the success of targeted ultrasound in finding a correlate and the reported percentage varies from 23 to 67%.[10,11,12,13,14] In a study of 519 patients with suspicious MRI findings by Meissnitzer et al, a sonographic correlate was found in 56% of cases.[12] Ultrasound was more successful in finding a correlate for masses than for nonmass enhancement. Among masses, 62% were identified with ultrasound, whereas only 31% of nonmass enhancement was found and for nonmass enhancement measuring 10 mm or less, a sonographic correlate was found in only 13%. Other factors that increased the likelihood of finding a sonographic correlate were increased size and malignant versus benign histology. The information as to which lesions are most likely to have an ultrasound correlate can help guide which MR-detected lesions are best managed by going directly to MRI-guided biopsy. The results of a number of studies on targeted ultrasound after MRI are summarized in ▶ Table 8.2.

Whereas finding a sonographic correlate to an MR finding is often straightforward, occasionally the lesion seen on MR and the lesion found on targeted ultrasound is not the same. When performing the targeted ultrasound, care should be taken to ensure the quadrant, size, shape, and appearance of the lesion as well as the distance from the nipple are similar between the two studies. In addition, a clip should always be placed at the time of sonographic biopsy. If the results of the biopsy are benign and felt to be concordant, a follow-up MRI should be performed to confirm correlation between the two findings. In the study by Meissnitzer et al, of 80 cases of benign, concordant ultrasound-guided biopsy for an MR finding, the two lesions did not correlate in 10 (12.5%) and 5 proved to be cancers (▶ Fig. 8.1).[12] In another study of 218 ultrasound-guided biopsies done for MR findings, the false-negative rate was 26% because of the lack of concordance between the two examinations.[15]

Table 8.2 Targeted ultrasound (US) for suspicious magnetic resonance imaging findings

Author (year)	N	Seen on US: total	seen on Us: malignant[a]	Not seen on US: total	Not seen on US: malignant[a]
LaTrenta et al (2003)[10]	93	21 (23%)	9 (43%)	55 (77%)	10 (14%)
DeMartini et al (2009)[11]	167	76 (46%)	27 (36%)	91 (54%)	20 (20%)
Meissnitzer et al (2009)[12]	519	290 (56%)	87 (34%)	229 (44%)	34 (19%)
Abe et al (2010)[13]	202	115 (51%)	33 (28%)	87 (49%)	11 (13%)
Destounis et al (2009)[14]	182	1280 (70%)	39 (32%)	54 (30%)	8 (16%)

[a]Percentage of malignant of those that underwent biopsy (positive predictive value [PPV3]).

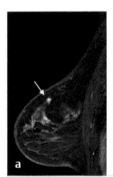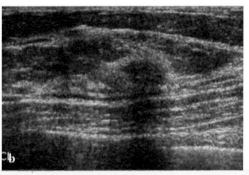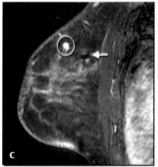

Fig. 8.1 Ultrasound–magnetic resonance imaging (MRI) correlation. (a) Showing sagittal postcontrast T1-weighted MRI showing 5-mm enhancing mass found on screening MRI (arrow). Targeted ultrasound revealed a hypoechoic mass thought to represent a sonographic correlate to the MR finding (b). Ultrasound-guided biopsy showed fibroadenomatoid change that was felt to be concordant. On follow-up MRI 6-months later (c), the signal void from the biopsy marker placed at the time of ultrasound biopsy (arrow) did not correspond to the original mass (circled) that was still present and larger. Subsequent MRI-guided biopsy revealed invasive ductal carcinoma.

Both of these studies emphasize the importance of careful correlation between ultrasound and MR findings and follow-up MR when biopsy results are benign and concordant in order to ensure accurate sampling of the lesion.

The optimal timing of the follow-up study has not been fully established. A case report suggested a strategy for correlation whereby a single noncontrast, non–fat-suppressed sequence is obtained immediately after the ultrasound-guided biopsy.[16] The follow-up MRI should take just a few minutes to perform and the signal void from the clip placed at the time of biopsy should be readily apparent and can confirm accurate sampling. However, if the lesion is surrounded by glandular or fibrous tissue rather than fat, correlation may be difficult without the administration of contrast (▶ Fig. 8.2). Depending on availability of the magnet, an immediate postbiopsy may not be logistically feasible. Also, it is unlikely that any reimbursement could be obtained for this single sequence. For most cases, doing a 6- to 12-month follow-up MRI for benign concordant ultrasound-guided biopsies for a suspicious finding on MR may be sufficient.

8.3 Before the Biopsy

8.3.1 Equipment

MRI-guided breast biopsies can be safely performed on either 1.5- or 3-T magnets and do not have to be done on the same field strength magnet used for the AB-MR examination. MRI-guided biopsies require devices that allow targeting of the lesion in the breast. The two types of devices are the compression grid and the pillar-and-post apparatus. These devices add on to the breast coil and are used to allow needle insertion into the appropriate location in the breast. Most allow access to the lateral and the medial surface of the breast simultaneously, allowing biopsy of multiple sites in a single breast. Some coils also allow simultaneous access to the lateral aspects of both breasts, allowing bilateral biopsies. If there are

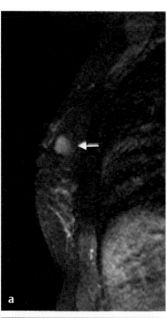
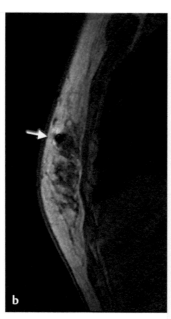
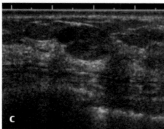

Fig. 8.2 Immediate postbiopsy imaging for concordance. Enhancing mass found on sagittal T1-weighted image (*arrow*, **a**). Targeted ultrasound showed mass that was thought to represent the correlate. Ultrasound-guided biopsy was performed and a clip placed (**b**). T1-weighted sequence without fat suppression done immediately after the ultrasound biopsy (**c**) shows the signal void from the biopsy marker clip (*arrow*) within the mass, confirming that the ultrasound finding was indeed the correlate.

bilateral lesions and one or both must be accessed from a medial approach, bilateral biopsies at the same time are not possible and must be done on separate visits.

Any of a variety of needles can be used with the targeting devices. Most are vacuum assisted and range from 7 to 14 gauge, though the most commonly used are 9 to 11 gauge. Some have automatic collection of the core specimen in a collection chamber; others require manual retrieval of the cores. All of the MRI needle devices have similar components. There is usually a nonmetallic sheath with centimeter markings that allows the lesion depth to be set, a sharp introducer that fits through the sheath, a needle guide, and a plastic obturator that allows scanning to confirm accurate location of the sheath (▶ Fig. 8.3). The actual sampling needle is then advanced through the sheath for tissue acquisition. As with any piece of equipment, the choice of which device and which needle to use is a matter of individual preference.

The reported time required to perform a single site MRI-guided biopsy is between 35 and 58 minutes.[4,17,18] Noroozian et al evaluated the time required for MRI-guided biopsies as a function of patient, lesion, and technical variables.[18] They reported that factors such as patient age, breast size, lesion size, mass versus nonmass enhancement, or lesion location were not associated with the length of time of the procedure. The only factor that affected procedure time was the presence of a breast imaging fellow in training which decreased duration of the biopsy. Despite the fact that image acquisition time is faster with 3-T magnets, they found no significant difference in procedure time for those done on 3-T compared to 1.5-T magnets.

Multiple sites and bilateral lesions will of course require more time. Liberman et al reported the average time of biopsy for a single lesion to be 35 and 65 minutes for two lesions.[4] Lehman et al had a mean time of 59 minutes when multiple lesions in one breast were biopsied and 64 minutes when bilateral biopsies were done.[17] For a single lesion, scheduling 1 hour of magnet time should be sufficient.

Because the time of lesion visualization is limited due to washout and enhancement of surrounding parenchyma over time, it is advisable to be thoroughly familiar with the location and appearance of the lesion and to plan the approach prior to the procedure. During a full MR examination, a sequence in the plane orthogonal to the plane of acquisition of the dynamic series is often obtained. For example, if the postcontrast sequences are obtained in the axial plane, a single sagittal sequence is sometimes performed as the last sequence allowing visualization of a lesion in two planes. With the abbreviated protocol, imaging in only one scan plane is acquired and therefore, it may be advisable to reformat in the orthogonal plane prior to the biopsy for optimal procedure planning. This is particularly important if the biopsy is performed manually, without the aid of computer targeting software.

8.3.2 Patient Preparation and Consent

Informed consent should obviously be obtained prior to all procedures. In speaking with the patient, the risk of bleeding and hematoma formation should be discussed. Another potential

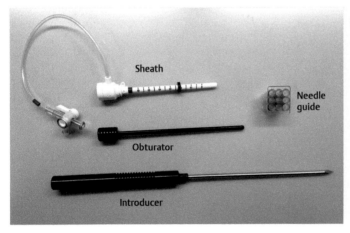

Fig. 8.3 Typical needle biopsy setup.

Sheath

Needle guide

Obturator

Introducer

complication is infection, which can occur days or weeks after the procedure. It is not customary to administer prophylactic antibiotics prior to breast biopsy procedures in general.

Fortunately, serious complications from core biopsy procedures in general are relatively rare. There are very few reported cases of complications secondary to MRI-guided core biopsies, but in one review of core biopsies in general that included nearly 29,000 lesions, the incidence of serious complications was less than 1%.[19] This study reported an incidence of hematoma requiring treatment of 0.09% and infections requiring antibiotics in 0.15%. The biopsies in these studies were performed with 11- and 14-gauge needles, whereas MRI-guided biopsies are often done with 9-gauge needles, and it is possible that the incidence of significant bleeding with MRI-guided biopsies may be higher than with smaller gauge needles, though still relatively low. Perlet et al, in a multicenter study, had serious bleeding in 3 out of 334 (0.9%) biopsies that required surgical intervention and 1 case of infection requiring antibiotics.[2]

It is common practice to stop anticoagulation, particularly with warfarin or chronic low-dose aspirin prior to the procedure. However, there is some evidence that MRI-guided biopsies can be safely performed even in women who are anticoagulated. In a very small series of core biopsies of 18 lesions in women on anticoagulation with warfarin (11 lesions), aspirin (6 lesions), or heparin (1 lesion), no clinically important complications occurred.[20] Similarly, Somerville et al reported on a series of core biopsies done on 200 women on aspirin (180), warfarin (16), and other nonsteroidal anti-inflammatory drugs (NSAIDs; 4).[21] They compared these women to 855 others who were not on anticoagulation and found that there was a statistically significant incidence of bruising among the anticoagulated group (34 vs. 26.5%, $p = 0.035$), but there was no significant difference in the occurrence of hematomas. Therefore, both of these studies concluded that core biopsies can be done on women on anticoagulation especially if stopping the anticoagulant is associated with more risk than the risk of hematoma formation. However, if there is no compelling reason to continue anticoagulation, both of the authors continue to stop medication before the procedure. If warfarin cannot safely be stopped, it is advisable to check the international normalized ratio (INR) prior to the biopsy to be certain it is not above therapeutic range.

A potential complication unique to MRI-guided procedures is reaction to gadolinium. All women having MRI-guided biopsies have already had an MRI examination with gadolinium, presumably without untoward effect, but there is no guarantee that a reaction will not occur. However, serious reactions to gadolinium-based contrast are uncommon. In one series of over 158,000 examinations in which gadolinium was administered intravenously, only 15 cases required treatment, with the most common reaction being hives.[22]

The presence of an implant is not an absolute contraindication to MRI-guided biopsy although it can make the procedure technically challenging. When there is an implant present, mention of the remote possibility of inadvertent implant rupture should be included in the consent process.

In obtaining consent, it is advisable to include a discussion of clip placement and the need for a postprocedure mammogram to document the location of the clip. Some women object to the presence of a clip, but when presented with the reasons a clip is needed, the advantages of clip placement and the lack of documented complications associated with clips, patients usually agree to have one placed. It should be explained that a clip is needed in case more tissue needs to be removed should the biopsy results come back showing malignancy or a high-risk lesion and without the clip, localization will need to be done with MR guidance rather than with mammographic guidance, which is faster, easier, and more comfortable for the patient. In addition, if the biopsy results are benign and concordant, the clip indicates the site of biopsy on future MR examinations. Because AB-MR is done for screening, it is likely that these patients will have repeated MRIs and having documentation of the location of the biopsy may be helpful in future interpretation. The fact that the patient will not experience pain or any other untoward effects from the clip, that it will not set off metal detectors, and that it will not interfere with future MRI examinations can be stressed. It is quite helpful to have an actual clip available to show patients who are concerned to show how tiny they are.

It is good practice to tell the patient when the pathology results are likely to be available and to formulate a plan for conveying the results. Ideally, the results should be given to the patient by the radiologist who performs the procedure as he/she is the person who can best assess concordance of imaging and pathology. A management recommendation should always be included in the report of the procedure and ideally, this recommendation should be conveyed directly to the patient.

8.3.3 Technique

The steps in performing MRI-guided core biopsies are listed here with details of each step outlined in this section.

- Position patient.
- Do pre- and postcontrast T1-weighted sequences. This can be in the axial or sagittal plane, depending on your equipment.
- Target the lesion.
- Cleanse the skin and apply local anesthetic.
- Position the sampling sheath using the introducer.
- Replace the metal introducer with the plastic obturator and scan to be sure position of the sheath is correct.
- Obtain samples.
- Scan with obturator in place to be sure the lesion was successfully sampled.
- Place a clip.
- Scan to confirm clip placement (optional).
- Do mediolateral (ML) and craniocaudal (CC) mammograms to confirm clip location.

8.3.4 Patient Positioning

It is important that the patient's breast be positioned in the breast coil by an experienced technologist. Not uncommonly, technologists who are trained in performing MRI examinations are not accustomed to positioning the breast. When starting an MR biopsy program, if the MRI technologists are not familiar with the principles of positioning, technologists from the breast imaging section can assist initially in positioning the patient for MRI biopsies until the MRI technologists are comfortable and proficient in performing this task. Positioning for MRI biopsies is similar to positioning for stereotactic breast biopsies. Medial and lateral breast tissue should be pulled into the coil as much as possible and the nipple should be in profile and be in the center of the coil. Having a well-trained technologist position the patient can make the difference between allowing access to a lesion in a difficult position in the breast and having to cancel the procedure. Time and effort should also be given to making the patient as comfortable as possible before starting in order to minimize the possibility of movement during the biopsy.

If an implant is present, implant displacement technique should be utilized to move the implant out of the compression device as much as possible, just as is done with stereotactic biopsy positioning (▶ Fig. 8.4). This may not be possible, however, depending on the location of the implant and the degree of capsule formation. If the implant cannot be safely displaced away from the lesion, core biopsy may not be possible. In these cases, MRI-guided needle localization can be attempted.

The compression grid or pillar and post should be placed at the surface of the breast closest to the lesion, either lateral or medial. Some devices allow a grid to be placed simultaneously on both the lateral and medial surfaces and this can be advantageous if the lesion is close to the midline. Under compression, the lesion may move closer to one side of the breast or the other and having the ability to approach from either the medial or the lateral surface can minimize the amount of tissue that needs to be traversed in order to reach the target.

Compression should be firm enough to prevent lesion movement but not overly tight so as to compromise blood flow and potentially prevent adequate lesion visualization. In a study of the effect of breast compression evaluating the degree of compression applied during biopsy procedures and comparing lesion size in the noncompressed to the compressed breast, Khouli et al showed that

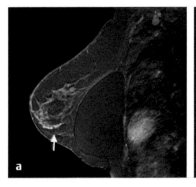
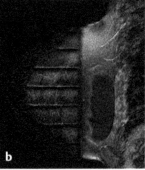

Fig. 8.4 Postcontrast T1-weighted image shows nonmass enhancement in a woman with an implant (**a**). Magnetic resonance imaging guided biopsy was recommended. The patient was positioned in the biopsy coil with the implant displaced, allowing for successful sampling (**b**).

the degree of compression applied during the biopsy procedure varied considerably and that the application of compression resulted in decreased accuracy in lesion size determination and visibility.[23]

In most cases, intravenous contrast will need to be administered not only to locate the lesion, but also to be certain the lesion is still enhancing. It is advantageous to obtain a precontrast sequence to be certain positioning is correct, fat suppression is adequate, and the fiducial marker can be seen. In addition, having a precontrast sequence allows for subtraction to be performed if necessary for optimal visualization of the abnormality. Power injection is not absolutely necessary because analysis of kinetics is not performed. However, it is important to be able to inject without the need to move the patient out of the bore of the magnet in order to minimize the possibility of patient movement.

8.3.5 Targeting

All of the commercially available computer-aided detection (CAD) systems have automated targeting software that simplifies identifying the location of a lesion in the breast. However, just as pilots need to know how to fly airplanes manually despite the availability of autopilot, it is important for radiologists who do MRI-guided biopsies to know how to target without the aid of the software programs in case of computer or software malfunction.

For targeting using the fenestrated grid, a fiducial marker must be placed and included on the images. With the automated software programs, fiducials are either built into the compression device or placed at a preset location within the fenestrated compression grid. For the automated systems,

scanning can be performed in either the sagittal or the axial plane. The lesion is marked and the software determines the appropriate opening in the fenestrated grid, the appropriate opening in the needle guide, and the depth of the lesion from the skin surface (▶ Fig. 8.5).

For manual targeting with the fenestrated grid, commercially available markers that are visible on T1-weighted images can be used, although a simple vitamin E capsule will suffice. For manual targeting, the marker is placed in any one of the grid openings. Scanning is done either in the sagittal plane or in the axial plane with reconstruction. On the MRI workstation, the lesion is marked on sagittal images and the slices are scrolled back to the grid to determine the appropriate opening to use. This represents the x- and y-axis location of the lesion. For the depth (z-axis) location, the number of slices between the skin surface and the lesion is determined and then multiplied by the slice thickness to get the depth. For example, if the skin surface is seen on image 3 and the lesion on image 13, there are 10 slices between the two. If the slice thickness is 3 mm, the lesion is 10×3 or 30 mm from the skin. These steps are illustrated in ▶ Fig. 8.6.

The orientation of the patient on the workstation is different from the orientation of the patient in the magnet. In order to ensure that the correct grid opening is used, all of the compression grid device manufacturers have printed sheets that allow indication of which opening should be targeted (▶ Fig. 8.7). This is then brought into the magnet room and flipped to reflect the patient's orientation.

For the pillar-and-post device, either the axial or the sagittal plane can be used. With the patient in

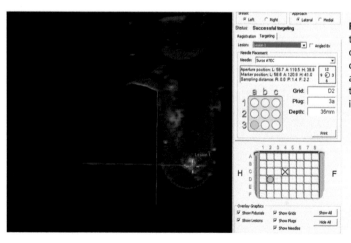

Fig. 8.5 Targeting with computerized targeting software. The lesion is found on either axial or sagittal sequence. A cursor is placed on the lesion and the appropriate grid opening, opening in the needle guide, and depth are indicated.

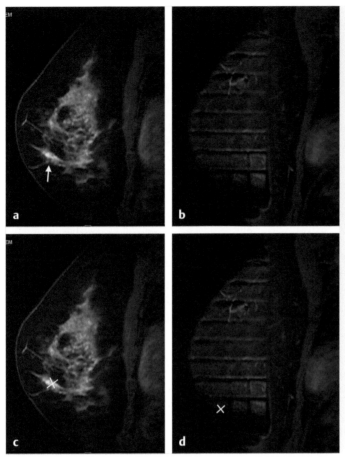

Fig. 8.6 Manual targeting using the fenestrated grid. T1-weighted image showing nonmass enhancement for which magnetic resonance imaging guided biopsy was recommended (*arrow*, **a**). Patient is placed in grid and the slice number showing the grid is noted (**b**). The lesion is then found and the slice number is determined. The number of slices between the grid and the lesion multiplied by the slice thickness indicates the depth of the lesion, or z-axis. A cursor is placed on the lesion (**c**) and the sequence is scrolled back to the grid. The grid opening with the cursor (*cross*) determines the x- and y-positions of the lesion (**d**).

compression, the pillar is set to zero location in both the x- and y-axes. A fiducial marker is placed and imaging is performed. The fiducial is marked on the slice on which it appears and a reference line is placed on the workstation. The x-axis (horizontal) location is determined by the number of slices between the fiducial and the lesion multiplied by the slice thickness. The vertical location (y-axis) is calculated as the distance from the lesion to the fiducial reference line. Once the x- and y-axis locations are determined, the fiducial is removed, and the patient rescanned to be certain that the location of the pillar is correct. The z-position is measured as the distance from the skin surface to the lesion to determine the depth. These steps are illustrated in ▶ Fig. 8.8.

8.3.6 Tissue Acquisition

Once targeting is accomplished, the skin at the targeted site is cleansed with antiseptic solution, usually iodine and/or alcohol. A skin wheal is then raised and superficial anesthesia is administered using approximately 2 or 3 mL of 1% Lidocaine without epinephrine. Additional deep anesthesia is often given using an additional 6 to 8 mL of 1% Lidocaine with epinephrine. If there is a contraindication to the use of epinephrine, Lidocaine without epinephrine can be used instead. If desired, a skin nick can be made with a scalpel with a no. 11 blade. This step is optional given the tip of the introducer is quite sharp. However, the wound from the scalpel nick is linear rather than a puncture and may heal with less of a scar. Once the needle guide is in place in the grid, the skin surface cannot be seen, so if a skin nick is made, the tip of the introducer should be put into the nick before the needle guide is placed in order to avoid having a separate wound.

The introducer is then pushed into the breast to the preset depth on the sheath. A twisting motion while pushing can help to avoid displacing the

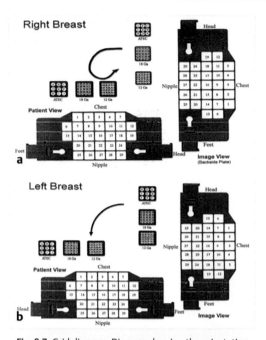

Fig. 8.7 Grid diagram. Diagram showing the orientation of the image on the workstation for the right breast **(a)** and left breast **(b)**. The location of the lesion is marked on the diagram which is brought into the magnet and rotated to reflect the patient's orientation in the breast coil allowing accurate localization. Four separate diagrams should be available, one for each breast from a lateral approach and one for each breast from a medial approach.

lesion ahead of the tip. When the sheath is at the appropriate depth, the introducer is removed and replaced with the obturator. The patient is then placed back into the bore of the magnet and a sequence to confirm accurate placement is performed. If scanning in the sagittal plane, the last slice showing the signal void of the obturator should be at the center of the lesion. In the axial plane, the tip of the obturator should be at the center of the lesion (▶ Fig. 8.9).

Once the sequence confirming accurate positioning of the introducer sheath is done, the patient is slid out of the magnet, the obturator removed, and the needle device placed through the sheath. The optimum number of cores to be obtained has not been firmly established but in most instances, six cores with a 9-gauge vacuum-assisted device should be sufficient. At that point, the obturator is again put into the sheath, the patient slid back into the magnet, and a sequence to confirm adequate sampling of the lesion obtained (▶ Fig. 8.10). Occasionally, because of patient or lesion movement, additional cores need to be obtained and for this reason, the needle assembly should be kept sterile while confirmatory imaging is performed.

After adequate sampling has been achieved, a clip is placed. Scanning after clip placement to document successful clip deployment is often not useful because the clip is obscured by biopsy changes. Usual postprocedure wound care is given

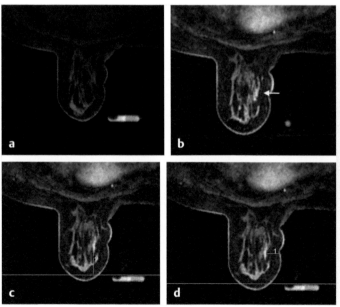

Fig. 8.8 Manual targeting using the pillar-and-post device. The location of the slice showing the fiducial is noted **(a)**. The slice showing the lesion (*arrow*) is then found **(b)** and the number of slices between the lesion and the fiducial is multiplied by the slice thickness to indicate the x-axis location. A reference line is placed on the slice with the fiducial and the distance between this line and the lesion indicates the y-axis location **(c)**. Finally, the distance from the lesion to the skin determines the depth, or z-axis **(d)**.

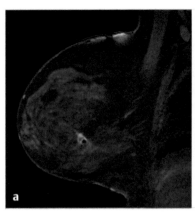
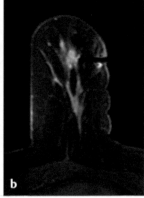

Fig. 8.9 Confirmation of accurate positioning of biopsy sheath. On sagittal imaging, the deepest imaging showing the signal void from the obturator should be in the center of the lesion, as is shown here **(a)**. On axial imaging, the end of the obturator, which marks the center of the sampling trough, ideally should be positioned near the center of the lesion **(b)**.

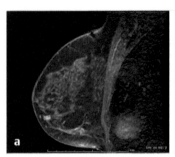
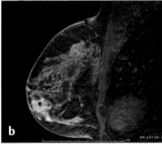

Fig. 8.10 Postbiopsy confirmation of accurate sampling. **(a)** The targeted lesion on prebiopsy image. **(b)** The immediate postbiopsy image showing biopsy change at the site of the lesion.

and the site compressed until all bleeding stops. Steri-Strips are applied and the patient is brought to the mammography suite for a two-view mammogram consisting of ML and CC views to document clip placement. After the mammogram, a pressure dressing is applied and postbiopsy instructions given.

8.4 Challenges and Pitfalls

There are several challenging situations and pitfalls associated with performing MRI-guided core biopsies. Many are similar to those encountered with other types of image-guided procedures, particularly stereotactic biopsies where positioning is similar. One situation that is unique to MRI-guided procedures is nonvisualization of the target at the time of biopsy. This has been reported to occur in 8 to 14% of cases for which MRI-guided biopsy is attempted. This may occur because the original lesion represented background parenchymal enhancement that no longer enhances, presumably due to hormonal effects, or because enhancement is hampered by compression. Hefler et al reported nonvisualization in 13% (37/291) of scheduled biopsies,[24] Perlet et al reported an incidence of

12.5% in a multicenter study,[5] and in the series by Brennan et al 8% (74/911) were not seen at the time of attempted biopsy.[25] In that series, abnormalities occurring in dense breasts and in those with moderate or marked background enhancement were more likely to be canceled than those in nondense breasts or those with minimal or mild background. There was no difference in cancellation as a function of mass versus nonmass enhancement patterns in their series.

When a lesion is not seen at the time of attempted biopsy, delayed imaging can be performed in order to allow visualization. If the lesion is not seen on delayed sequences, subtraction can sometimes reveal the lesion. If these steps still do not show the abnormality, there are two choices in terms of management. If the location of the lesion is readily identified despite the lack of enhancement and if the originally seen lesion is particularly suspicious, biopsy can be performed based on landmarks. More often, however, the biopsy will be canceled and follow-up performed. This is because most lesions that show nonvisualization at the time of biopsy do not need to be sampled and will not be seen on subsequent MRI examinations. However, follow-up should always be performed for these cases as occasionally, a cancer will not be seen at the time of attempted biopsy but will reappear on follow-up (▶ Fig. 8.11). In the series by Hefler et al, follow-up MRI was done in 29 cases within 6 months of cancelation and the lesion was gone in 25 but again seen in 4.[24] In 3 of the 4, subsequent biopsy yielded malignant results. In the report by Brennan et al, 29% (17/58) of cases undergoing follow-up imaging at a mean of 12 months reappeared.[25] At the time the study was published, none were malignant on biopsy or further follow-up, but one case went on to mastectomy for an ipsilateral cancer and ductal carcinoma in situ (DCIS) was found in the same quadrant as the initially seen abnormal enhancement. In addition, since the publication of this study, two cases have been identified on follow-up imaging that were indeed cancers. The optimal timing of the follow-up examination has not been definitively determined. Hefler et al suggest very short interval follow-up of 4 to 24 hours.[24] Brennan et al recommend short-interval follow-up imaging but do not specify a time interval. Despite this recommendation, the median time to follow-up in their series was 12 months.[25]

8.4.1 Posterior Lesions

Posterior lesions pose a challenge to core biopsy because abnormalities located close to the chest wall may not be able to be included in the grid, precluding the ability to perform the biopsy. When this occurs, the padding on the coil can be removed to provide an additional centimeter or so of posterior tissue. The patient can be oblique so that more posterior tissue is pulled into the grid.

Finally, the needle can be positioned anterior to the lesion and preferential sampling toward the chest wall can sometimes allow successful biopsy. There are some instances, however, where the lesion cannot be accessed and in those cases, MRI-guided wire localization can usually be accomplished.

8.4.2 Medial Lesions

Because of the design of the breast coils and biopsy grids, access to lesions located medially in the breast is often more limited than for those in the lateral aspect. Therefore, lesions located in the posterior medial breast may not be accessible enough to allow biopsy. If the abnormality is just medial to midline and the breast is of sufficient thickness, approaching the lesion from the lateral surface of the breast may be possible. Another potential solution to posterior medial lesions is to position the breast to be biopsied in the opposite breast coil. For example, if the lesion is in the medial left breast, putting the left breast in the right breast coil makes the medial surface of the right breast accessible (▶ Fig. 8.12). The limitation to this technique, however, is that the positioning is awkward for the patient and can be very uncomfortable. In addition, this technique can be used only on slim to average-sized women because when the patient is obliqued, she may not fit into the bore of the magnet.

8.4.3 Thin Breasts

The breast in compression must have sufficient thickness to accommodate the length of the sampling trough as well as the dead space at the end

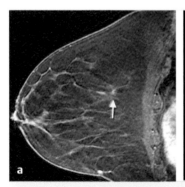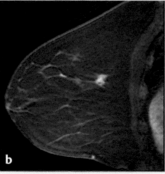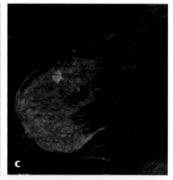

Fig. 8.11 Lesion nonvisualization at time of attempted biopsy. Screening magnetic resonance imaging (MRI) in a woman at high risk for breast cancer shows an irregular focus of enhancement (*arrow*) new from prior studies (**a**). At the time of attempted MRI-guided biopsy, no lesion was visualized (**b**). The biopsy was canceled and short interval follow-up was recommended. On follow-up MR, the lesion is again seen, increased in size (**c**). Biopsy showed invasive ductal cancer.

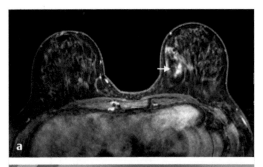

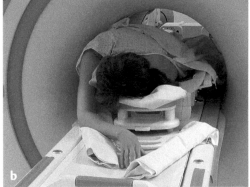

Fig. 8.12 Positioning for medial lesions in the breast. (a) Nonmass enhancement in the medial left breast is seen (*arrow*) for which MRI-guided biopsy was recommended. (b) The patient was positioned with her left breast in the right breast coil opening, making the medial aspect of the left breast accessible.

of the needle. This thickness will vary according to the device used but in general, requires approximately 2 cm beyond the center of the lesion. Unlike most stereotactic devices that indicate with an audible signal if breast thickness is insufficient and that performing the procedure will risk penetrating the opposite surface of the breast, MRI coils do not have this built-in safeguard. If the breast thickness is too thin to accommodate the standard needle, there are needles with shorter troughs and blunt tips that will not pierce the skin of opposite surface of the breast.

8.4.4 Superficial Lesions

If a lesion is located just under the skin, the calculated *z*-position, which places the center of the sampling trough at the center of the lesion, may result in a portion of the trough being outside the skin. Biopsy cannot be performed because the vacuum will not be functional. In these cases, the

needle with the shorter sampling trough can be used. The trough can be buried just beneath the skin allowing successful sampling. Care must be taken, however, to completely bury the trough. If a small amount of the trough is at the skin surface rather than just beneath it, a bit of skin can be taken with each core, resulting in a large skin defect at the end of the procedure that may require sutures to close and result in a suboptimal cosmetic effect. Because the skin entrance site is obscured by the needle guide, it can be difficult to be certain the trough is buried. It is possible to insert the sheath freehand without the needle guide as long as care is taken to insert the sheath with a straight trajectory. The sheath can be supported by a tape sling while scanning is performed.

8.4.5 Lesion Displacement

Occasionally, especially when the breasts are very dense or when a mass is located in fatty breasts, the lesion can be displaced by the introducer. In many cases, accurate targeting can be achieved by repositioning the introducer, but in some cases, the lesion will continue to be pushed away. When this happens, the needle can be positioned as close as possible to the lesion and preferential sampling in the direction of the abnormality can be performed (▶ Fig. 8.13).

8.4.6 Needle Too Deep in the Breast

A common pitfall in MRI-guided breast biopsies is placing the needle beyond the lesion (▶ Fig. 8.14). This can occur especially when the breast tissue is dense and pressure must be applied to advance the introducer to the desired depth. With some systems, the stopper placed on the sheath to mark the depth of the lesion is not firmly fixed and can be moved inadvertently. It is important to note the position of the posterior aspect of the depth stopper and take care not to go beyond this setting.

8.5 Postprocedure Management

8.5.1 Clip-Related Issues

Once tissue acquisition is completed, a sequence is performed to confirm adequate sampling and a clip is placed. Commonly, air is introduced to the

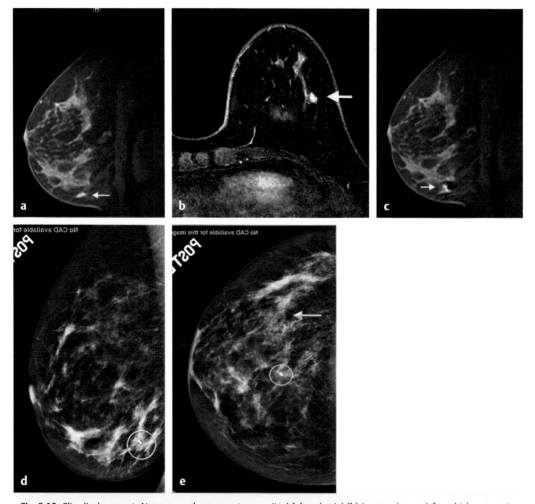

Fig. 8.13 Clip displacement. Nonmass enhancement on sagittal (**a**) and axial (**b**) images (*arrows*) for which magnetic resonance imaging guided biopsy was performed. Postbiopsy sagittal sequence indicates accurate sampling of the lesion (**c**, *arrow*). Postbiopsy mediolateral mammogram shows clip in accurate location (**d**). Craniocaudal mammogram (**e**), however, shows the clip (*circle*) medially displaced from the biopsy site (*arrow*).

biopsy site during the procedure and this obscures visualization of the clip. Scanning after clip placement is not often helpful. Before the procedure, mammograms should be reviewed to determine if other clips are present and if so, it is desirable to use a different-shaped clip if possible. Also, if multiple sites in one breast are biopsied, different-shaped clips should be placed and careful note of which shape clip marks which lesion should be included in the procedure report.

Pressure is applied until bleeding stops and a mammogram is performed to document clip placement and ascertain the location of the clip in relation to the biopsy site. As with stereotactic biopsies, some of the problems encountered with the clip include nondeployment and clip displacement. Clip nondeployment can be due to defective equipment or incomplete deployment with inadvertent withdrawal of the clip along with the clip introducer. There is also a case report of disappearance of a clip that was confirmed to be present on post-MRI biopsy mammograms but was not seen at the time of subsequent wire localization.[26] Usually, failure of the clip to deploy is not discovered until the patient has the postprocedure mammogram. At that point, it is not practical to put the patient back in the magnet to place another clip. Ultrasound can be used to try to identify the

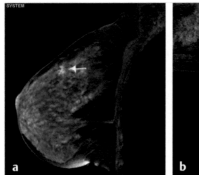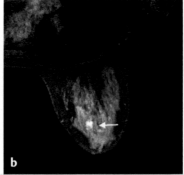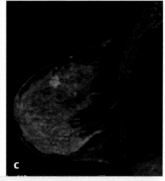

Fig. 8.14 False-negative magnetic resonance biopsy. Sagittal postcontrast T1-weighted image from a screening magnetic resonance imaging (MRI) examination shows irregular nonmass enhancement (**a**, *arrow*). Postbiopsy image suggests accurate sampling (**b**). Histology showed usual ductal hyperplasia, sclerosing adenosis, and focal fibrosis, felt to be concordant. Follow-up MRI 6 months later shows the lesion to still be present and larger (**c**). Repeat biopsy showed invasive ductal carcinoma.

biopsy site and a clip placed under ultrasound guidance. Alternatively, if pathology results indicate the need for excision, localization under MRI guidance can be performed.

Clip displacement away from the biopsy site occurs not uncommonly, usually along the z-axis due to either the accordion effect or migration of the clip along the needle tract (▶ Fig. 8.15). The frequency with which this occurs on MRI has not been established but has been reported with stereotactic biopsies.[27] This is why the postprocedure mammogram is crucial after clip placement. If the clip is displaced from the expected location, the direction and amount of displacement can be included in the biopsy report. If surgical excision is necessary, often, a combination of clip location and landmarks can allow for mammographic rather than MRI localization despite displacement.

8.5.2 Imaging-Pathologic Concordance

Proper performance of an MRI-guided biopsy does not end with tissue acquisition. It is essential that the radiologist who performs the procedure obtain the pathology result and correlate the results with the imaging features of the biopsied lesion to determine concordance. Discordant results should be followed by repeat biopsy, usually by surgical excision. As with any other image-guided biopsy, discordant results are those in which benign histology is obtained but the imaging appearance is highly suspicious. It also occurs

when the pathology does not explain the imaging finding, such as when benign fatty breast tissue is obtained for an enhancing mass. Finally, cases in which technical challenges suggest that the lesion may not have been adequately sampled and benign, nonspecific pathology is obtained may be considered discordant.

Concordance determinations are more difficult for MRI-guided procedures than for other stereotactic or ultrasound-guided biopsies because a large number of nonspecific benign entities including normal parenchyma and fibrocystic change can enhance on MR. Additionally, unlike other image-guided biopsies where specimen radiographs can be obtained or real-time confirmation of adequate sampling is possible, it is often difficult on MRI-guided biopsies to be certain, despite acquiring postbiopsy sequences, that the lesion was actually sampled.

The reported rate of discordant results at MR biopsy ranges from < 1 to 7%.[3,8,28]

The upgrade rate for discordant MR biopsies has been reported to be higher than for other image-guided procedures, perhaps due to the fact that MRI is generally done only on high-risk women. Lee et al found 7% of their cases were discordant and of those, the upgrade rate was 30%.[28] Orel et al encountered discordant results in 2 of 86 biopsies (2%) with cancer diagnosed at excision in both of these cases.[3] Mahoney had a 5% discordant rate among 55 lesions, but none were upgraded to malignancy.[6] Clearly, all discordant cases should undergo repeat biopsy or surgical excision.

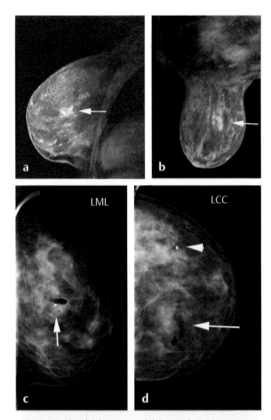

Fig. 8.15 Clip displacement. **(a)** Sagittal postcontrast image showing focal nonmass enhancement (*arrow*) that underwent magnetic resonance imaging guided biopsy. **(b)** Axial image showing the nonmass enhancement in the medial aspect of the breast (*arrow*). **(c)** Left mediolateral postbiopsy mammogram. The clip (*arrow*) appears to be in accurate position in the biopsy cavity. **(d)** Left craniocaudal postbiopsy mammogram shows the clip (*arrowhead*) to be laterally displaced from the biopsy site (*arrow*). This was likely due to the accordion effect. The biopsy report should clearly state that the clip is displaced.

8.5.3 High-Risk Lesions

High-risk lesions are those that are themselves benign but that can be found in association with malignancy. They often require surgical excision after core biopsy to be certain a sampling error has not occurred. High-risk lesions encountered on MRI-guided biopsies are the same as those found with other image-guided biopsies and include atypical ductal hyperplasia (ADH), lobular neoplasia including lobular carcinoma in situ (LCIS) and atypical lobular hyperplasia (ALH), radial scar, papilloma, and fibroepithelial lesions that could represent possible phyllode tumors. High-risk lesions have been reported to occur in 5 to 22% of MRI-guided biopsies, most performed with 9- to 11-gauge needles.[2,3,4,6,7,8,17,29,30,31] The reported upgrade rate ranges from 13 to 57%, but these numbers are difficult to interpret because the definition of what constituted a high-risk lesion and criteria for which lesions underwent subsequent excision after MR biopsy varied considerably among the different studies.[32]

As with other image-guided core procedures, the most common high-risk lesion encountered on MR biopsy in most series is ADH. The reported upgrade rate is generally 30 to 50%[7,8,17,29,30,31] and most, though not all, practices will excise ADH when found on core biopsy. In the majority of cases, upgrade from ADH on core is to DCIS, but invasive cancer can also sometimes be found. Lieberman et al reported finding ADH in 6% (15/237) of their series of MRI-guided biopsies with an upgrade of 38%, all DCIS.[29] Lourenco et al found high-risk lesions in 21.5% of 446 MR biopsies, and an overall upgrade rate of 23%.[31] Among the cases of ADH in their series, the upgrade was 32% and included both DCIS and invasive disease.

The management of other high-risk lesions besides ADH is more controversial. There are very few reported cases of LCIS and ALH specifically encountered on MR biopsies, and some series combine the two entities under the term lobular neoplasia. At least two studies, however, have reported upgrades of single cases of LCIS or ALH to invasive cancer after MRI-guided core biopsy[6,8] and in one series, four of eight cases of lobular neoplasia were upgraded to malignancy (DCIS in three and invasive cancer in one).[30] The literature on LCIS and ALH when encountered on ultrasound or stereotactic biopsy reports very variable upgrade rates and not all practices routinely excise classic LCIS or ALH after core biopsy. When atypical or pleomorphic LCIS is encountered, however, data support surgical excision because of an upgrade rate of 25%.[33]

There is also quite a bit of confusion and disagreement as to management of papillary lesions encountered on core biopsies, including MRI-guided procedures. Whereas most papillary lesions with atypical features warrant excision, some do not consider benign papillomas to be high-risk lesions and do not routinely excise them.[32] Brennan et al specifically studied papillomas diagnosed on MRI-guided core biopsies.[34] They encountered 75 papillomas among 1,487 biopsies (5%), 25 with atypia and 50 without. At surgery, there was an overall upgrade rate of 6%, all to DCIS. Two of the upgrades were in papillomas with atypia for an upgrade rate of 9% and 2 in papillomas without atypia for an upgrade rate of 5%. The difference between these two rates was not statistically significant and the authors conclude that both papillomas with and those without atypia found on MRI-guided core biopsy warrant surgical excision.

To date, no cases of upgrade of radial scar on MRI-guided core biopsies have been reported, but the numbers are small.[32] Unfortunately, no clinical or imaging factors have been identified that can predict which high-risk lesions are more likely to be upgraded.[30,35] Because there are no clear guidelines for many of the so-called lesions encountered on MRI-guided core, a reasonable strategy would be to manage the results of these biopsies in the same manner as stereotactic or ultrasound-guided biopsies. It has been suggested, however, that the upgrade rate of high-risk lesions found on MRI-guided core may be higher than that of stereotactic biopsies, perhaps because of the fact that MRI is reserved for women at high risk for breast cancer.[29,35] The incidence of high-risk lesions and upgrade rates from several studies are summarized in ▶ Table 8.3.

8.5.4 False-Negative Biopsies and Follow-Up Imaging

A concern with any type of biopsy is the possibility of false-negative results. This is particularly true for MRI-guided biopsies where bleeding at the biopsy site, lesion washout, or enhancement of the surrounding tissue may make it impossible to be certain that the lesion was adequately sampled. The rate of false-negative MRI biopsies has been reported to be 0 to 4.5%.[2,36,37,38,39,40]

The lack of real-time confirmation of successful sampling and the reported incidence of false-negatives emphasizes the importance of performing follow-up imaging. What is still to be definitively determined is the optimum follow-up interval. Bahrs et al performed follow-up within 24 to 48 hours of 299 MRI biopsies thought to be technically successful.[40] They found that 18 lesions were actually missed and on re-biopsy 13 were malignant. No other false negatives were subsequently identified and the authors state that the false-negative rate can be reduced to zero by doing such short interval imaging. Hauth et al also advocate performing repeat imaging to confirm sampling within 24 hours.[36] In their series of 29 cases, 1 was seen at 24-hour follow-up to have been missed and was DCIS on excision.

Doing very short interval follow-up within 1 or 2 days may not be logistically feasible for many patients or practices and insurers may not reimburse for a repeat examination so soon after the biopsy. Li et al evaluated the timing of follow-up MRI after benign concordant MRI biopsies.[41] They found 4 cancers initially missed among 177 lesions detected on follow-up imaging. They also found that doing the follow-up before 6 months was not helpful and recommend that all MRI biopsies with benign concordant results have follow-up at 6 months. A consensus statement on MRI-guided biopsy issued by an interdisciplinary European panel recommended follow-up of benign, concordant cases in 6 to 12 months.[42]

Table 8.3 Incidence and upgrade of high-risk lesions

Author (year)	N	high risk	Upgrade[a]
Perlet et al (2002)[2]	334	17 (5%)	3 (18%)
Mahoney (2005)[6]	55	7 (13%)	4 (57%)
Liberman et al (2007)[29]	98	10 (10%)	3 (30%)
Orel et al (2006)[3]	85	18 (21%)	3 (17%)
Han et al (2008)[7]	150	21 (14%)	4 (25%)
Crystal (2011)[30]	161	31 (19%)	13 (50%)
Rauch (2012)[8]	218	37 (17%)	5 (14%)
Lourenco (2014)[31]	446	96 (22%)	16 (23%)

[a]Percentage upgrade of cases undergoing biopsy (positive predictive value [PPV3]).

8.5.5 MRI-Guided Needle Localization

Image-guided core biopsy has a number of advantages over open surgical biopsy, including less morbidity, time, and cost, and is the preferred method for evaluating nonpalpable breast abnormalities. There are some situations, however, when needle localization will be performed rather than core biopsy and this is true for MRI findings as well. Localization and excision is necessary for biopsy of a lesion that is not accessible to MRI-guided core, including lesions that are posterior, in the axillary tail, close to the nipple, superficial, or located in very thin breasts or adjacent to an implant that cannot be displaced (▶ Fig. 8.15). There is more latitude in needle placement for localization than for core biopsy, so many lesions that are inaccessible to core can be successfully localized. Other situations where wire localization and surgery may be more appropriate than core include cases in which MRI-guided core yielded malignancy or a high-risk lesion that needs excision, but no clip was placed or if the clip was significantly displaced. In addition, when MRI is done for extent of disease, bracketing of the extent of enhancement on MRI may be desired.

The technique of targeting for MRI-guided needle localization is identical to that of core biopsy with the exception that after the depth of the lesion is calculated, an additional 1.5 to 2 cm should be added to account for the width of the needle guide and to allow the wire to traverse the lesion. It is not essential that the needle guide be used and for some lesions, particularly those close to the nipple or those located closer to the chest wall than the grid, freehand placement can be done. Morris et al, in a series of 101 MRI-guided needle localization procedures, reported a malignancy rate of 31% and a mean procedure time of 31 minutes.[43]

There are specially designed MRI-compatible needles and wires that look identical to the ones routinely used. The difference, however, is that the wire is more fragile and may be more apt to be transected or to break if pulled too forcefully. In the series of 101 MRI-guided needle localizations reported by Morris et al, complications included retained wire fragments in 2 cases and breakage of the wire in 1.[43] Surgeons should be cautioned about the increased fragility of the wire. Specimen radiographs after MRI-guided location will not usually show the lesion but can be helpful in documenting that the entire distal portion of the localizing wire was removed.

8.6 Conclusion

In order for any screening program to be successful in decreasing mortality, the ability to obtain tissue for definitive diagnosis is essential. There are a number of steps in performing high-quality biopsy procedures that include preprocedure patient preparation, technique of tissue acquisition, concordance assessment, and appropriate postbiopsy management and follow-up. Each of these steps is equally important and one way of ensuring quality work is to audit results, tracking not only PPV, but also complications, rate of high-risk lesions, rate of upgrade, and false negatives. In doing this, outcomes from screening with abbreviated MRI can be optimized to maximally benefit patients.

8.7 References

[1] Breast MRI Accreditation. www.acr.org/Quality-Safety/Accreditation/BreastMRI. Accessed July 22, 2015

[2] Perlet C, Heinig A, Prat X, et al. Multicenter study for the evaluation of a dedicated biopsy device for MR-guided vacuum biopsy of the breast. Eur Radiol. 2002; 12(6):1463–1470

[3] Orel SG, Rosen M, Mies C, Schnall MD. MR imaging-guided 9-gauge vacuum-assisted core-needle breast biopsy: initial experience. Radiology. 2006; 238(1):54–61

[4] Liberman L, Bracero N, Morris E, Thornton C, Dershaw DD. MRI-guided 9-gauge vacuum-assisted breast biopsy: initial clinical experience. AJR Am J Roentgenol. 2005; 185(1):183–193

[5] Perlet C, Heywang-Kobrunner SH, Heinig A, et al. Magnetic resonance-guided, vacuum-assisted breast biopsy: results from a European multicenter study of 538 lesions. Cancer. 2006; 106(5):982–990

[6] Mahoney MC. Initial clinical experience with a new MRI vacuum-assisted breast biopsy device. J Magn Reson Imaging. 2008; 28(4):900–905

[7] Han B-K, Schnall MD, Orel SG, Rosen M. Outcome of MRI-guided breast biopsy. AJR Am J Roentgenol. 2008; 191(6):1798–1804

[8] Rauch GM, Dogan BE, Smith B, Liu P, Yang WT. Outcome analysis of 9-gauge MRI-guided vacuum-assisted core needle breast biopsies. AJR Am J Roentgenol 2012 198(2):292–299

[9] Manion E, Brock JE, Raza S, Reisenbichler ES. MRI-guided breast needle core biopsies: pathologic features of newly diagnosed malignancies. Breast J. 2014; 20(5):453–460

[10] LaTrenta LR, Menell JH, Morris EA, Abramson AF, Dershaw DD, Liberman L. Breast lesions detected with MR imaging: utility and histopathologic importance of identification with US. Radiology. 2003; 227(3):856–861

[11] Demartini WB, Eby PR, Peacock S, Lehman CD. Utility of targeted sonography for breast lesions that were suspicious on MRI. AJR Am J Roentgenol. 2009; 192(4):1128–1134

[12] Meissnitzer M, Dershaw DD, Lee CH, Morris EA. Targeted ultrasound of the breast in women with abnormal MRI findings for whom biopsy has been recommended. AJR Am J Roentgenol. 2009; 193(4):1025–1029

[13] Abe H, Schmidt RA, Shah RN, et al. MR-directed ("Second-Look") ultrasound examination for breast lesions detected

initially on MRI: MR and sonographic findings. AJR Am J Roentgenol. 2010; 194(2):370–377

[14] Destounis S, Arieno A, Somerville PA, et al. Community-based practice experience of unsuspected breast magnetic resonance imaging abnormalities evaluated with second-look sonography. J Ultrasound Med. 2009; 28(10):1337–1346

[15] Sakamoto N, Tozaki M, Higa K, Abe S, Ozaki S, Fukuma E. False-negative ultrasound-guided vacuum-assisted biopsy of the breast: difference with US-detected and MRI-detected lesions. Breast Cancer. 2010; 17(2):110–117

[16] Monticciolo DL. Postbiopsy confirmation of MR-detected lesions biopsied using ultrasound. AJR Am J Roentgenol. 2012; 198(6):W618–620

[17] Lehman CD, Deperi ER, Peacock S, McDonough MD, Demartini WB, Shook J. Clinical experience with MRI-guided vacuum-assisted breast biopsy. AJR Am J Roentgenol. 2005; 184 (6):1782–1787

[18] Noroozian M, Gombos EC, Chikarmane S, et al. Factors that impact the duration of MRI-guided core needle biopsy. AJR Am J Roentgenol. 2010; 194(2):W150–157

[19] Bruening W, Fontanarosa J, Tipton K, Treadwell JR, Launders J, Schoelles K. Systematic review: comparative effectiveness of core-needle and open surgical biopsy to diagnose breast lesions. Ann Intern Med. 2010; 152(4):238–246

[20] Melotti MK, Berg WA. Core needle breast biopsy in patients undergoing anticoagulation therapy: preliminary results. AJR Am J Roentgenol. 2000; 174(1):245–249

[21] Somerville P, Seifert PJ, Destounis SV, Murphy PF, Young W. Anticoagulation and bleeding risk after core needle biopsy. AJR Am J Roentgenol. 2008; 191(4):1194–1197

[22] Hunt CH, Hartman RP, Hesley GK. Frequency and severity of adverse effects of iodinated and gadolinium contrast materials: retrospective review of 456,930 doses. AJR Am J Roentgenol. 2009; 193(4):1124–1127

[23] El Khouli RH, Macura KJ, Kamel IR, Bluemke DA, Jacobs MA. The effects of applying breast compression in dynamic contrast material-enhanced MR imaging. Radiology. 2014; 272 (1):79–90

[24] Hefler L, Casselman J, Amaya B, et al. Follow-up of breast lesions detected by MRI not biopsied due to absent enhancement of contrast medium. Eur Radiol. 2003; 13(2):344–346

[25] Brennan SB, Sung JS, Dershaw DD, Liberman L, Morris EA. Cancellation of MR imaging-guided breast biopsy due to lesion nonvisualization: frequency and follow-up. Radiology. 2011; 261(1):92–99

[26] Bourke AG, Peter P, Jose CL. The disappearing clip: an unusual complication in MRI biopsy. BMJ Case Rep. 2014; 2014: bcr2014204092

[27] Esserman LE, Cura MA, DaCosta D. Recognizing pitfalls in early and late migration of clip markers after imaging-guided directional vacuum-assisted biopsy. Radiographics. 2004; 24 (1):147–156

[28] Lee J-M, Kaplan JB, Murray MP, et al. Imaging histologic discordance at MRI-guided 9-gauge vacuum-assisted breast biopsy. AJR Am J Roentgenol. 2007; 189(4):852–859

[29] Liberman L, Holland AE, Marjan D, et al. Underestimation of atypical ductal hyperplasia at MRI-guided 9-gauge vacuum-

assisted breast biopsy. AJR Am J Roentgenol. 2007; 188 (3):684–690

[30] Crystal P, Sadaf A, Bukhanov K, McCready D, O'Malley F, Helbich TH. High-risk lesions diagnosed at MRI-guided vacuum-assisted breast biopsy: can underestimation be predicted? Eur Radiol. 2011; 21(3):582–589

[31] Lourenco AP, Khalil H, Sanford M, Donegan L. High-risk lesions at MRI-guided breast biopsy: frequency and rate of underestimation. AJR Am J Roentgenol. 2014; 203 (3):682–686

[32] Heller SL, Moy L. Imaging features and management of high-risk lesions on contrast-enhanced dynamic breast MRI. AJR Am J Roentgenol. 2012; 198(2):249–255

[33] Chivukula M, Haynik DM, Brufsky A, Carter G, Dabbs DJ. Pleomorphic lobular carcinoma in situ (PLCIS) on breast core needle biopsies: clinical significance and immunoprofile. Am J Surg Pathol. 2008; 32(11):1721–1726

[34] Brennan SB, Corben A, Liberman L, et al. Papilloma diagnosed at MRI-guided vacuum-assisted breast biopsy: is surgical excision still warranted? AJR Am J Roentgenol. 2012; 199(4): W512–519

[35] Strigel RM, Eby PR, Demartini WB, et al. Frequency, upgrade rates, and characteristics of high-risk lesions initially identified with breast MRI. AJR Am J Roentgenol. 2010; 195 (3):792–798

[36] Hauth EA, Jaeger HJ, Lubnau J, et al. MR-guided vacuum-assisted breast biopsy with a handheld biopsy system: clinical experience and results in postinterventional MR mammography after 24 h. Eur Radiol. 2008; 18(1):168–176

[37] Raher L, Wisner D, Chang B, Esserman L, Hylton N, Joe B. False Negatives Found on Follow-Up MRI after Benign Concordant MRI-Guided Breast Biopsies (abstr). Chicago, IL: RSNA; 2011

[38] Friedlander L, Lee C, Comstock D, Morris E, Dershaw DD. Frequency of Unsuspected Missed Lesions and False-Negative Rate at MRI-Guided Core Biopsy (abstr). Chicago, IL: RSNA; 2011

[39] Shaylor SD, Heller SL, Melsaether AN, et al. Short interval follow-up after a benign concordant MR-guided vacuum assisted breast biopsy—is it worthwhile? Eur Radiol. 2014; 24(6):1176–1185

[40] Bahrs SD, Hattermann V, Preibsch H, et al. MR imaging-guided vacuum-assisted breast biopsy: reduction of false-negative biopsies by short-term control MRI 24–48 h after biopsy. Clin Radiol. 2014; 69(7):695–702

[41] Li J, Dershaw DD, Lee CH, Kaplan J, Morris EA. MRI follow-up after concordant, histologically benign diagnosis of breast lesions sampled by MRI-guided biopsy. AJR Am J Roentgenol. 2009; 193(3):850–855

[42] Heywang-Kobrunner SH, Sinnatamby R, Lebeau A, Lebrecht A, Britton PD, Schreer I, Consensus group. Interdisciplinary consensus on the uses and technique of MR-guided vacuum-assisted breast biopsy (VAB): results of a European consensus meeting. Eur Rad 2009;72:289–294

[43] Morris EA, Liberman L, Dershaw DD, Kaplan JB, LaTrenta LR, Abramson AF, Ballon DJ. Preoperative MR imaging-guided needle localization of breast lesions. AJR Am J Roentgenol 2002;178(5):1211–1220

Index

Note: Page numbers set **bold** or *italic* indicate headings and figures, respectively.

AB-MR Interpretation Overview

- Goal of AB-MR interpretation is to maintain high sensitivity and specificity
- In order to minimize false positives and short term follow ups, it is fundamental to identify only findings that are truly unique to the background parenchymal enhancement (BPE)
- Biopsy and short-term follow up should be reserved for lesions ≥3 mm in size

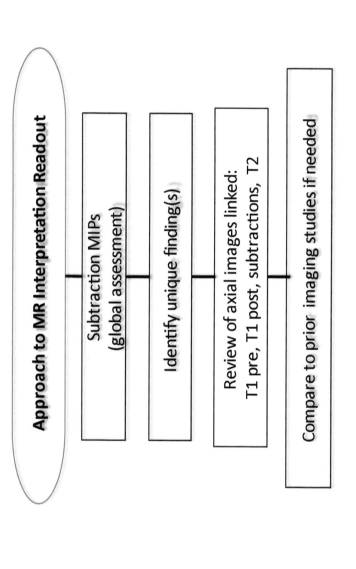

Approach to MR Interpretation Readout

Subtraction MIPs (global assessment)

Identify unique finding(s)

Review of axial images linked: T1 pre, T1 post, subtractions, T2

Compare to prior imaging studies if needed

Algorithm 1 Approach to magnetic resonance interpretation readout. (Reproduced with permission of the SBMR.)

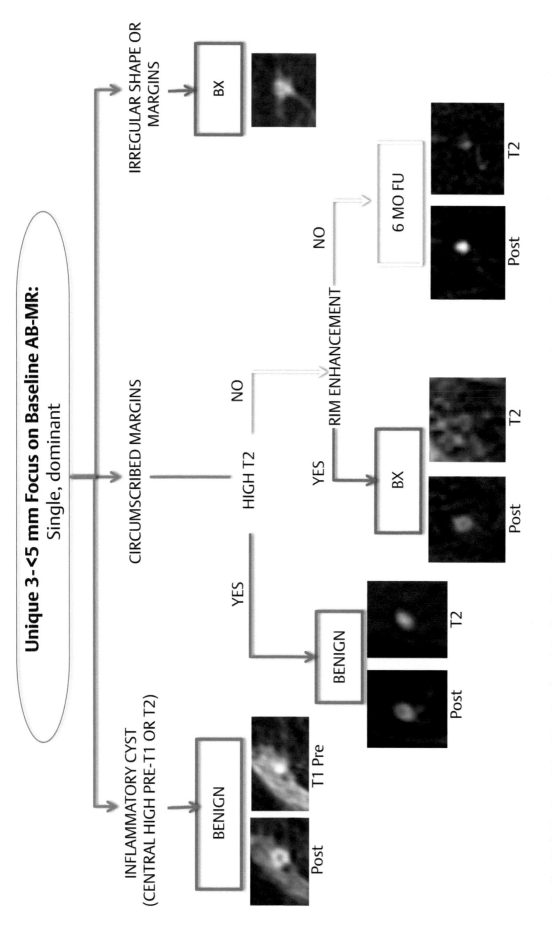

Algorithm 2 Interpretation guidelines for a unique focus on baseline abbreviated breast magnetic resonance imaging (AB-MR). (Reproduced with permission of the SBMR.)

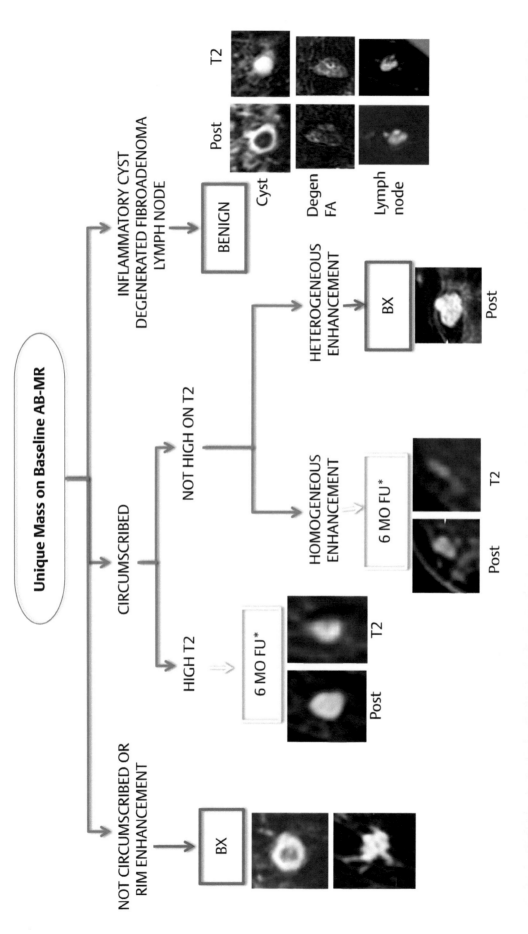

Algorithm 3 Interpretation guidelines for a unique mass on baseline abbreviated breast magnetic resonance imaging. (Reproduced with permission of the SBMR.)

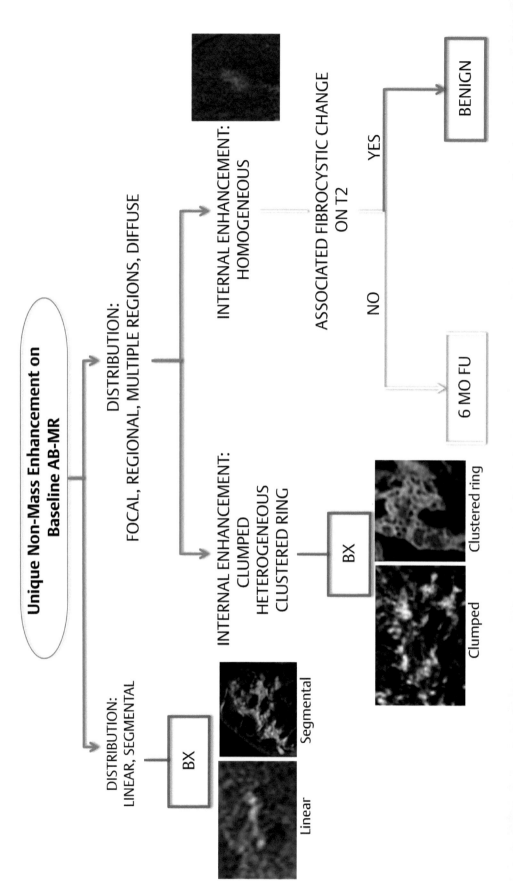

Algorithm 4 Interpretation guidelines for unique nonmass enhancement on baseline abbreviated breast magnetic resonance imaging. (Reproduced with permission of the SBMR.)